THE PATIENT MULTIPLE

Wyse Series in Social Anthropology

Editors:
James Laidlaw, William Wyse Professor of Social Anthropology, University of Cambridge, and Fellow of King's College, Cambridge
Maryon McDonald, Fellow in Social Anthropology, Robinson College, University of Cambridge
Joel Robbins, Sigrid Rausing Professor of Social Anthropology, University of Cambridge, and Fellow of Trinity College, Cambridge

Social Anthropology is a vibrant discipline of relevance to many areas – economics, politics, business, humanities, health and public policy. This series, published in association with the Cambridge William Wyse Chair in Social Anthropology, focuses on key interventions in Social Anthropology, based on innovative theory and research of relevance to contemporary social issues and debates. Former holders of the William Wyse Chair have included Meyer Fortes, Jack Goody, Ernest Gellner and Marilyn Strathern, all of whom have advanced the frontiers of the discipline. This series intends to develop and foster that tradition.

THE PATIENT MULTIPLE

An Ethnography of Healthcare
and Decision-Making in Bhutan

Jonathan Taee

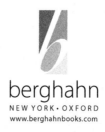

berghahn
NEW YORK · OXFORD
www.berghahnbooks.com

Published in 2017 by
Berghahn Books
www.berghahnbooks.com

Library of Congress Cataloging-in-Publication Data

Names: Taee, Jonathan, author.
Title: The patient multiple : an ethnography of healthcare and decision-making
    in Bhutan / Jonathan Taee.
Description: New York : Berghahn Books, 2017. | Series: WYSE series in social
    anthropology ; volume 4 | Includes bibliographical references and index.
Identifiers: LCCN 2016053205 (print) | LCCN 2016055843 (ebook) | ISBN
    9781785333941 (hardback : alk. paper) | ISBN 9781785333958 (ebook)
Subjects: LCSH: Medical Anthropology--Bhutan. | Traditional medicine--
    Bhutan. | Traditional medicine--Technological innovation--Bhutan.
Classification: LCC GN296.5.B47 T34 2017 (print) | LCC GN296.5.B47 (ebook)
    | DDC 306.4/61095498--dc23
LC record available at hips://lccn.loc.gov/2016053205

British Library Cataloguing in Publication Data

A catalogue record for this book is available
from the British Library.

ISBN 978-1-78533-394-1 (hardback)
ISBN 978-1-78533-395-8 (ebook)

This book is dedicated to the patients
and healthcare practitioners of Bhutan.

May you long find hope and healing from one another.

Contents

Maps, Illustrations and Figures

Maps

Illustrations

Figures

An online collection of colour photography accompanying
this book is available at: www.jonathantaee.com

Acronyms

I have avoided using acronyms in the body of the text. Acronyms are used in parenthesised references and are spelled out in their full form on first appearance.

BBC	British Broadcasting Corporation
BBS	Bhutan Broadcasting Service
BHU	Basic Health Unit
BST	Bhutan Stretchable Time
DDC	Dzongkha Development Commission
DRA	Drug Regulatory Authority, Royal Government of Bhutan
DVED	Drug, Vaccines and Equipment Division, Royal Government of Bhutan
FTM	Faculty of Traditional Medicine
INR	International Normalised Ratio
MLHR	Ministry of Labour and Human Resources, Royal Government of Bhutan
MoAF	Ministry of Agriculture and Forests, Royal Government of Bhutan
MoH	Ministry of Health, Royal Government of Bhutan
MSP	Menjong Sorig Pharmaceuticals (Formally known as PRU)
NSB	National Statistics Bureau, Royal Government of Bhutan
NITM	National Institute of Traditional Medicine
NTMH	National Traditional Medicine Hospital
OCC	Office of the Census Commission, Royal Government of Bhutan
PRU	Pharmaceutical Research Unit (Now called MSP)
RGoB	Royal Government of Bhutan
WHO	World Health Organisation

Notes on Language, Transliteration, Transcription and Translation

Dzongkha (*rdzong kha*) is the national language of Bhutan, one of twenty-seven active languages. It is spoken by approximately 160,000 people, most of whom live in the western part of the country (Ethnologue, ISO 639-3, 2013). The second most common non-English language is Sharshop (*shar phyogs pa*), also known as Tshangla Lo (*thangs la lo*, Driem 1998: 27–29), used primarily in the east of Bhutan; however, this particular language is further broken down into different dialects and subgroups (see Phuntsho 2013: 51–62). My informants would often clump these eastern languages together using the umbrella term Sharshop, literally translated as '[the language of the people of] the eastern direction.' Dzongkha has roots in Classical Tibetan, known in Bhutan as Chöke (*chos skad*). These languages share the same script, yet they are definitively different. George van Driem, one of the leading experts on Dzongkha and other Himalayan languages, notes, "The relationship between Dzongkha and Chökê in Bhutan is reminiscent of the role Latin used to play as the language of learning in Mediaeval France where the spoken language had long since evolved into a language different from that spoken by the ancient Romans" (1991: 4).

The relationship between Dzongkha and modern Tibetan is complicated historically, linguistically and politically, yet a cursory introduction is necessary to present a sound methodology for handling Dzongkha in this book.

The connection between the two languages can be found in the historical use of Chöke as a written language. Before the mid-twentieth century Dzongkha was a spoken language only; until the mid-1960s, Chöke was the only written language in Bhutan (Phuntsho 2013: 53). More recent records show that only in the 1960s was Chöke replaced in favor of a new orthographic form of Dzongkha in schools (Driem and Tshering 1998: 7–8), alongside the adoption of English for the core curricula. Throughout the 1900s as Bhutan's government and institutions started to form, they too implemented Dzongkha as the main language of communications. In 1971, the third King Jigme Dorji Wangchuk commanded the further development of Dzongkha grammar and pushed the National Assembly to adopt it as the national language of Bhutan (Kinga 2009: 248). In

2008, the Constitution of the Kingdom of Bhutan (Royal Government of Bhutan, RGoB 2008: 1) was formally published, officially listing Dzongkha as the national language. Therefore, as a standardized language it is relatively new, and although more people are speaking it with greater fluency due to its use in media, government, education and other sectors, there remain many in Bhutan who still cannot speak it.

Linguistically, Dzongkha is considered a South Tibetan language with close relation to 'J'umowa' spoken in the Chumbi Valley in Tibet (Driem 2004: 294). Although modern-day spoken Dzongkha and Tibetan are in most cases mutually unintelligible, the literary and orthographic forms are closely related due to their influences from liturgical Chöke (Driem 1998: 4–5). Like Tibetan, Dzongkha uses the *ucen* (*dbu can*) script for formal documents and the *joki* (*mgyogs yig*) script for shorthand (Allen 2012: 325–34). While the script is the same, some orthographic spellings are pronounced differently in Dzongkha and Tibetan. These differences are discussed below as I argue for how to deal with phonetic transcription.

In today's political context, the Bhutanese government and its institutions are keen to identify the autonomous and distinctive nation-state of Bhutan, within which Dzongkha as a unique language plays an important part. Thus there is a strong effort to separate Dzongkha from its Tibetan ancestry concerning its contemporary application and historiographies. Meanwhile, many academics and linguists are keen to reconnect the two, looking for narrative trails between them. These pushes and pulls require a level of reflexiveness for those looking to engage with the Dzongkha language in presenting ethnographic evidence. To what extent does one 'Tibetanize' Dzongkha or conversely isolate it away from Tibetan and the masses of literature that accompany it? In the face of such challenges, I have attempted to use systems of transliteration and transcription that allow accessibility to the language and pronunciation for non-specialist readers and render the contemporary spelling and phonetic use of Dzongkha into a resource cross-referenceable to other ethnographic work on origins of both Bhutanese and Tibetan languages.

While the Dzongkha Development Commission (DDC) has done extensive work to standardize the use of Dzongkha and its transliteration into romanization and translation into English (see for example DDC 2010), much variance in linguistic methodology persists in academic, institutional and commercial publications. Seldom do authors outline their approach to Dzongkha. There are different transliteration and transcription options available to those working with Dzongkha, for example George van Driem's (1991) 'Guide to Official Dzongkha Romanization', which focuses on transcription rather than orthographic transliteration. This method uses a linguistic system of conversion close to those used in Chinese and Southeast Asian languages, rendering terms like 'village' (གཡུས) as *ü*. Unfortunately such systems are challenging for nonlinguistic trained readers to glean the correct pronunciation; for example, an English reader would most likely render a more accurate pronunciation from the spelling of 'village' as *yül*.

Due to the relative inaccessibility of Driem's transcription method, I have preferred the use of David Germano and Nicholas Tournadre's (2003) 'THL Simplified Phonetic Transcription of Standard Tibetan', which renders Dzongkha terms close if not perfectly to their intended pronunciation, making it easier for readers to follow the text with accurate voicing. However, phonetic transcriptions are always a 'reconstruction' of language and therefore provide an imperfect system, requiring some reflexive explanation. There are instances in Dzongkha where the pronunciations of the orthographic forms do not match exactly those rendered by the THL Phonetic method. Driem's (1998) language-learning book, entitled *Dzongkha*, offers the most comprehensive guide to the correct pronunciation of orthographic forms. For this book, there are two important instances where the THL Phonetic method must be amended to allow for correct Dzongkha pronunciation.

The first is with the syllable *rgya*. THL Phonetic Transcription gives the sound *gya* as pronounced in Tibetan. In spoken Dzongkha this syllable takes the sound *ja*.

The second is the suffix syllable *ga*, for example from the term *srog*, meaning vital life force. THL Phonetic renders the suffix as *k*, and thus *srog* becomes the phonetic term *sok*. However, in spoken Dzongkha, it is more accurate to render the suffix *ga* as a *g*, thus rendering the example term *sog*.

All non-English terms, except for people and place names, are italicized and presented in this simple phonetic transcription. Names of places and people are not italicized. All place names follow the English versions as declared by the Dzongkha Development Commission (1997).

On the first instance of a non-English term's use, the phonetic transcription is given, followed by a language marker when the language is not Dzongkha (Dz), such as Sharshop (Shr) or Tibetan (Tb). In instances when languages are being mixed together, I use the marker (Eng) to signify the use of English.

Also on first instance of use, the orthographic forms of the Dzongkha words follow in parentheses, using the Wylie transliteration method. For example, Bhutan is known locally as Druk Yül ('brug yul), meaning 'Land of the Thunder Dragon.'

Wylie as the orthographic transcription method is arguably the most suitable and widely consulted by academics and institutions working on Bhutanese topics using the Dzongkha language. Because Dzongkha is written in the same script as Tibetan, Wylie clearly and accurately identifies the spelling of Dzongkha terms. However, as noted earlier, it should be noted that the pronunciation of some of Dzongkha's orthographic forms differs from the Tibetan script, and therefore Wylie should be used for spelling only.

All terminology referencing medical practices, such as 'biomedical', 'traditional' and 'alternative', retain lowercasing, as does 'traditional medicine's' translation from the formal Tibetan terminology, *sowa rigpa* (Tb: *gso ba rig pa*). The titles *drungtsho* (*drung 'tsho*, traditional physician) and *menpa* (*sman pa*, traditional clinical assistant) retain lowercasing, following the English use of the term 'doctor'.

Drungtsho and *menpa* represent both their singular and plural forms and do not take a plural 's'. This resembles their actual use by my informants who would most commonly not pluralize these terms.

Dzongkha Reference Guide

The following Dzongkha terms are regularly used throughout the book. Although all terms are translated and described in the text itself, I include a short translation of each term here to offer the reader a quick reference point for local terminology.

Phonetic Transcription	Orthographic Transliteration	Description
ara	*a rag*	Home-distilled alcohol.
ba sha ka	*ba sha ka*	A particular medicinal plant species that grows in high-altitude locations in the Himalaya. Its Latin name is *Corydalis crispa* Prain.
chi pé men	*phyi pa'i sman*	Biomedicine in Bhutan, literally translated as 'modern medicine'.
Druk Yül	*'brug yul*	An additional name for Bhutan, often translated as 'the Land of the Thunder Dragon'.
drungtsho	*drung 'tsho*	A traditional-medicine physician of the institutionalized form of Bhutanese traditional medicine.
drukpa men	*'brug pa'i sman*	Literally translated means 'Bhutanese medicine', usually referencing *nang pé men*.
dü	*bdud*	Malevolent spirit, often not of the Buddhist tradition, usually living in the landscapes surrounding villages.
dug	*dug*	Poison.
dzongkha	*rdzong kha*	The national language of Bhutan.
dzongkhag	*rjong khag*	An administrative and juridical 'district', similar to a 'county', of which there are twenty.
gewog	*rged 'og*	A further sub-district of the larger *dzongkhags*, usually referring to a group of villages with an average area of 250 square kilometres, of which there are 205.

Phonetic Transcription	Orthographic Transliteration	Description
gho	*go*	The national male dress of Bhutan.
gomchen	*sgom chen*	A lay religious practitioner usually not attached to a monastic institution.
gyü zhi	*rgyud bzhi*	The original medical text of *sowa rigpa*.
ja né	*bya nad &* *rgya nad*	A complex and multilayered disease category or type, described in detail in chapter 4.
kira	*dkyi ra*	The national female dress of Bhutan.
la	*bla*	The vital life force, sometimes translated as 'soul'.
la tor	*bla stor*	An alternative practice of returning lost souls (*la*), sometimes translated as 'catching the fear' (Shr: *yong tsung ma*).
lam	*blam*	A religious practitioner usually attached to a monastic institution, commonly known in the West as a lama.
lha khang	*lha khang*	A Buddhist temple.
lho menjong	*lho sman ljongs*	An alternative name for Bhutan translated as 'the Southern Land of Medicinal Plants'.
mé tsak	*me tshag*	An alternative practitioner who burns skin using hot metal, often a piece of iron.
men	*sman*	Medicine.
men khap	*sman khab*	Syringe.
menpa	*sman pa*	A clinical assistant in the institutionalized traditional-medicine system.
Mongar	*mong sgar*	A major town in Eastern Bhutan that hosts the country's second largest hospital, Mongar Regional Referral Hospital.
nang pé men	*nang pa'i sman*	The term for 'traditional medicine' commonly used to describe the institutionalized practice of *sowa rigpa* in Bhutan. Literally translated as 'Buddhist medicine'.
né	*nad*	Disease or illness.
nep	*nad pa*	Sick person, patient.
ngag	*sngags*	Mantra.
ngan	*ngen*	Poison derived from ill luck or malevolent wishes usually from a neighbour or other human enemy.
ngultrum	*dngul kram*	The Bhutanese national currency, abbreviated to *nu*. The phonetic follows the Dzongkha Development Commission's official romanization of the term rather than the THL Phonetic method.

Phonetic Transcription	Orthographic Transliteration	Description
pawo	*dpa' bo*	Male spirit medium.
pamo	*dpa' mo*	Female spirit medium.
puja		A general name for a religious ritual, also known as *rim dro*. Originally a Hindi term used often in conversation in Bhutan.
ra jip kyap ni	*rwa 'jib rkyab ni*	An alternative practice known as 'cutting and sucking' when performed with a horn (*ra, rwa*). Also known more generally as *trak jip kyap ni*.
rim dro	*rim gro*	A religious ritual also known as a *puja*.
ru ta	*ru rta*	A medicinal plant where the root is of particular importance.
sharshop	*shar phyogs*	The second most widely spoken language in Bhutan, especially in the eastern regions. Literally, 'the eastern direction'.
sog	*srog*	The vital principle or life force, also known as la.
sowa rigpa	*gso ba rig pa*	Commonly translated as 'the art and science of Buddhist healing', also known as Tibetan medicine, traditional medicine and, in Bhutan, *nang pé men*. This is the institutionalized form of traditional medicine in Bhutan.
sung kü	*srung skud*	The colourful blessed strings worn to protect against negative karma and evil spirits. Literally translated as 'protective cord'.
sung ma	*srung ma*	Protective paper amulets often accompanying *sung kü*.
Thimphu	*thim phu*	The capital city of Bhutan.
trak jip kyap ni	*khrag 'jib rkyab ni*	The general term for an alternative practice known as 'cutting and sucking', also known as *ra jip kyap ni*.
tsechu	*tshe bcu*	A major festival type held all over Bhutan.
tsi	*rtsis*	An astrology reading.
tu	*mthu*	Ill luck, sometimes translated as 'black magic', having the power to cause illness, often created by ill-wishing humans.
yül	*yul*	Simplest translation renders a village, or cluster of houses. However, the spatial, social and structural complexity behind the translation to 'village' should be noted.
yül lha	*yul lha*	A village or territorial deity. As with the term *yül* this is a very simplified translation.

Acknowledgements

First and foremost I'd like to thank all the patients and their families who opened their lives, stories, experiences, vulnerabilities and hopes to this research project. Thank you for your unrelenting willingness to participate in this work. I dedicate this book to you.

I pay my respects to those patients who did not recover and sadly lost their lives over the course of writing this book. I remember Neyzang, the Mongar widow, and her late husband; the woman from a mountainside in Haa and the tiny baby in an intensive-care-unit incubator. I also remember Pema Dolma, whose generosity made Mongar a family village to me. Finally, I remember the brave two-year-old girl whose fighting breaths and loving parents were inspirations of life and love. I will not forget you.

I send a special thank you to Pema; Tshomo, Sonam and their healthy son; Dechen and her parents; Singye; Ugyen; Nima and Tshering, all of whom were central characters and inspiration to this ethnography.

Thank you also to all the doctors, nurses, health staff, *drungtsho, menpa,* alternative healers, administrators, clinical assistants and other practitioners nationwide that gave their lives to helping patients in the face of illness and suffering. I am humbled by your tireless efforts towards healing.

I would like to thank the Ministry of Health, the Minister of Health, and the Royal Government of Bhutan for accepting and welcoming my research project. I would also like to thank all other government institutions that aided in this research, including many ministries and institutions.

I'd like to thank Dr. Lungten Wangchuk and the Research Ethics Board for Health in helping design an ethically sound project. You are doing excellent work.

I'd like to send particular gratitude to the National Traditional Medicine Hospital, the Faculty of Traditional Medicine and Menjong Sorig Pharmaceuticals for hosting me and this project. Your openness and hospitality made this book possible. Thank you especially to Drungtsho Karma Gaylek, Drungtsho Dorji Nidup, Drungtsho Dorji Wangchuk, Drungtsho Tshering Tashi, Drungtsho Karma Ugyen, Menpa Tshering Wangchuk, Menpa Namgyel Lhendup, Menpa Thinley Pelshom, Drungtsho Kuenzang Wangchuk, Dean

Dophu, Kinga Jampel, Ugyen Dendup, Singye Wangchuk, Karma Wangchuk, Manu Singh, Sherab Tenzin, Ugyen Wangdi, Menpa Jigmi Thinley and all other *drungtsho, menpa*, lecturers, staff and traditional medicine producers. You are all inspiring in what you do.

Thank you to the entire Mongar Hospital and its staff for graciously hosting my long stay in Mongar. You run a challenging healthcare centre, and you do it with compassion and happiness. I'd like to particularly thank Drungtsho Wangdi Phuntsho and family, Drungtsho Nima Wangdi and family, Menpa Kuenzang Chofel and colleague, Dr. Tapas Gurung, Dr. Sonam Gyamtsho, Dr. Ugyen Thinley, Dr. Kezang Namgyel, Dr. Hoffman, Dr. Jit Darnel, Mr. Omar Pati, Mr. Phuntsho, Dr. Namsa Dorji, the paediatrician, Nurse Rinchen Peldon, Nurse Taranidhi Adhikari, Thinley Penjore, Tshering Phuntso and Indra Sharma.

Thank you everyone at the Jigme Dorji Wangchuck National Referral Hospital for taking the time to talk with me and let me walk your halls. Especially I'd like to thank Dr. Ngawang Tenzin, Dr. Chencho Dorji, Dasho Gado Tshering, Dr. Dechen Wangmo, Nurse Tandin Pemo, Dr. Trashi Tenzin, Dr. Stephen King, Dr. Wangmo, Dr. Phillips, Dr. Kinley, Dr. Nirola and Nurse Pema Dolma.

In the world of Dzongkha languages I'd like to send a huge thank you to Tenszin Jamtsho and Yeshi Lhendup. Tenzin, your lessons, patience and acumen for teaching made this book possible. Thank you so much. Yeshi, your continued support in translation was invaluable.

In other regions of Bhutan I'd also like to thank Mr. Tshetila, Haa Drungtsho and Doctor, Phuntsho Wangdi, Tandin in Haa, Mr. Bhattarai, Mr. Karma Pelden, Seemon, Sangay Dawa, all farmers and collectors in Lingshi, Mr. Passang in Lingshi and all the staff at Lhuntse, Trashiyangtse, Khaling, Trashigang, Bumthang, Thimphu, Punakha, Paro, Lingshi and Wangdue Phodrang health clinics.

I send love and thanks to many Bhutan friends, including Manny, Jen, Bena, Melissa, Ariel, Hilary, Kent, Korice, Chelsea, Thomas, G10, Karma T., Namgay W., Claire, Kasha, Simeran, Nate, Matthias, Choki, Letho and family, Choeki and Rabten Apartments, Dorji, Lam, Lama Shenphen, Manju, Dolma, Sonam and many more.

I send special thanks to Michael Rutland OBE for guiding my approach to Bhutan and offering much advice along the way. I will never fully know your efforts to bring my research to fruition. Thank you.

I also thank Dasho Ugen Tshechup, whose belief and support in me and the research was ever-present. I am thankful for all you did for me in Bhutan.

I would like to specially thank Dr. Francoise Pommaret for so much crucial insight, knowledge and wisdom shared before, after and during my research. You are an inspiration for this work.

There have been so many other academics and wise tutors along the way, to whom I owe a debit of gratitude. Thank you especially to Dr. Mancall, Dr. Laidlaw, Dr. McKay, Dr. Bayly, Dr. Lazar, Dr. Howe, Dr. Gay, Dr. Hunt, Dr.

Schrempf, Mr. Melgaard and Mr. Dorji. I also owe a debt of gratitude to a midwife and friend, Charlotte Mayou, who offered crucial advice on newborns and neonatal care. Also, a huge thank you to my PhD colleagues who have sweated, bled and read alongside me. Good luck to us all.

To my editors and readers, Dr. Samuel, Dr. McDonald, Alison, Peggitty and Riam, I owe you all so much. Thank you all for being so diligent, devoted and patient in reviewing and editing this book.

To Dr. Hildegard Diemberger, who supervised the PhD research on which this book is based, I lay at your feet in prostration. Thank you for your patience, persistence, detail, support and encouragement throughout this work.

To Lauren, it has been a tough ride. Thank you for sticking in there with me and supporting me in this calling. I love you. And to Elsie, my new and beloved daughter, thanks for being patient while I was busy finishing this book. Your arrival at its culmination is a blessing.

To my family, as always you have stood by me in everything I do. Thank you for your unrelenting and compassionate support.

This book, and the ethnography it presents, was made possible by multiple sponsors. I sincerely thank all of you for your vital support and dedication to this project. Thank you to the Schools Compensation Act Settlement Trust; Christ's College, University of Cambridge for multiple awards; British Association for South Asian Studies, Anthony Wilkin Fund; Frederik Williamson Fund; Ridgeway-Venn Travel Scholarship; Richards Fund; and the Board of Graduate Studies, University of Cambridge.

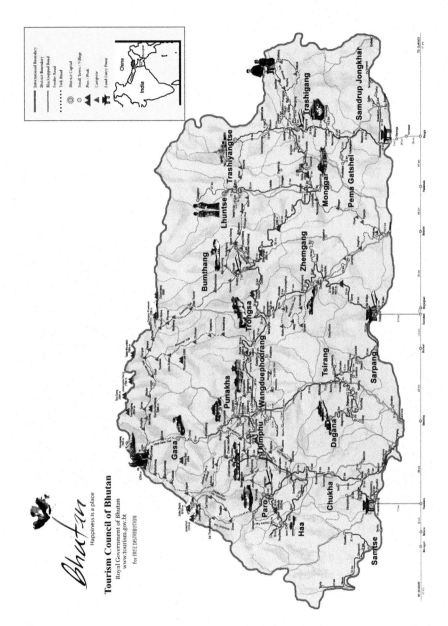

Map 0.1 Map of Bhutan: Cities, Towns and Roads. Source: Tourism Council of Bhutan, Royal Government of Bhutan, www.tourism.gov.bt

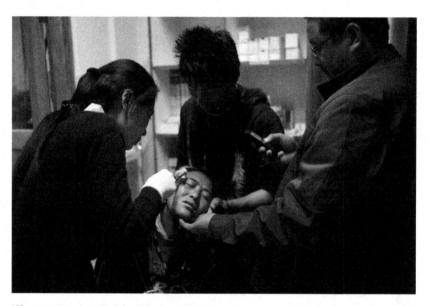

Illustration 0.1 Young Woman Receives Treatment, *Trashiyangtse Hospital, Mongar.* A young woman with an injured forehead visits the biomedical accident and emergency ward late at night in an eastern hospital. Her brother holds her head while the nurse cleans the wound.

Introduction

Orienting to Place and Practices

People all over the world fall ill and, in response, seek healing. Our experiences of illness in the context of healing practices, or our quest to find them, are a part of what it means to be human. This book is about what happens to people when sickness takes over their lives, inviting a complex set of understandings, reactions and experiences. It looks at these processes of suffering and healing in the context of Bhutan, a small landlocked country nestled in the Himalayan steppes, and the healthcare practices that are available throughout this country.

Bhutan is known as Druk Yül ('brug yul), Land of the Thunder Dragon. It is positioned between China and India, with Nepal to its west, from which it is separated by the Indian state of Sikkim. Its population of approximately 750,000 (World Bank 2015) live in the 38,394 square kilometres of valleys and steep slopes of the Himalayan Mountains, which descend from northern high altitudes to the southern low-lying planes of India (Ministry of Agriculture and Forests, MoAF 2013: 16). Over 70 percent of this land is covered in nationally protected forests (MoAF 2013: 16), a testament to Bhutan's progressive policies of wildlife and environmental conservation (see Kuyakanon Knapp 2015; RGoB 1995; Siebert and Belsky 2007; Buch-Hansen 1997). On the edges of these deep forests and steep mountain slopes, subsistence agriculturalists grow rice, chillies, potatoes and other vegetables, as well as keep a small amount of livestock. The agricultural labour force amounts to over 60 percent of the working population (Ministry of Labour and Human Resources, MLHR 2012: 20). The other 40 percent of the workforce are engaged in sectors like private business (19 percent, MLHR 2012: 20) and government (14 percent, MLHR 2012: 20), and live in the growing urban clusters, with Thimphu (thim phu), the capital, drawing the largest population (approximately eighty thousand, National Statistics Bureau, NSB 2005: 9).

Although significant gains were made in the past decade, Bhutan's economy remains one of the smallest in the world, with a 2012 GDP of USD$1.780 billion (World Bank 2015). Hydropower, collected and sold to India from a growing network of major dam projects, underpins the Bhutanese economy and offers a steady revenue stream for government administration.[1] While hydropower investment is intended to offer Bhutan greater economic self-sufficiency in the next ten to twenty years, the country's development projects have thus far received most of their financial support from international governments and institutions. These international revenue streams are channelled primarily into government-centralized projects, helping the state to build health, transport and hydropower infrastructure as well as to support other national development projects that have caused massive changes to the lives of Bhutanese citizens (Ura 2009c).

National development and poverty reduction have made remarkable progress in the last decade. Literacy rates climbing to 63 percent mark the growth in education and schools (NSB 2013c). Poverty rates below 12 percent that were over 23 percent in 2007 (NSB 2013a: 12) demonstrate household level changes, especially in rural areas that saw the most dramatic drop (30.9 percent in 2007 to 16.7 percent in 2012: 12).[2] Infant mortality rates have dropped from 102.9 in 1984 (Ministry of Health, MoH 2000a: 12) to 40.1 in 2010 (MoH 2010a: iii), highlighting progress in healthcare provision. Such gains have been framed by the government's dedication to its strategy of Gross National Happiness (GNH) – the pursuit of sustainable development, preservation of cultural values, conservation of the environment and good governance (Gross National Happiness Commission 2013: 5; Ura 2009a and 2009b). Commitment to GNH has led many Bhutanese officials to claim that while Bhutan has expedited its development over the last decade, it hasn't lost sight of its spiritual, environmental and social values, derived from Mahayana Buddhism, the predominant and guiding religion (see e.g. Al Jazeera 2010). Alongside such gains, Bhutan has developed into a democratic country, relatively stable and peaceful when compared with neighbours such as Pakistan or Myanmar. However, Bhutan is not without its political, social and economic problems, both past and present. There continue to be challenges facing the leaders and peoples of Bhutan; GNH simply offers a guiding policy for the decision-making process (see e.g. Wangyal 2001 and Brooks 2013).

One of the leading priorities of GNH and the development goals of Bhutan's governments and monarchs was the founding and proliferation of a national healthcare service that could offer free healthcare to patients nationwide. This effort began in the early 1900s thanks to the first king Ugyen Wangchuck (1907 to 1926), who hosted international doctors. Health services were then institutionalized as the Ministry of Health (MoH 2013b) in the 1960s and are still heavily under development today (C. Dorji 2009). The advent of health services has changed in dramatic ways the experiences of illness and suffering for all of Bhutan's population. There are still generations of elderly Bhutanese who remember the days when such services were not available and when sickness imposed a greater risk to life than it does today. One elderly patient answered my question about what happened when he fell ill as a young man: 'If you got sick, you got better. If not, you died.' Combined with other historical accounts of patient conditions (Melgaard and Dorji 2012: 72–74) and early reports of morbidity and life expectancy (MoH 1986: 17–20), we can assert that the success rates for curative practices in the early 1900s and before were not good, resulting in this man's matter-of-fact attitude towards illness, healing and death. Times have changed, but only recently. The last decade has seen a dramatic improvement in access to and quality of healthcare practices in both urban and rural locations. Patients now have diagnostic and treatment options. They are 'citizens' with the 'right' to 'services', all terms that are themselves the products of state-institution agendas. Learning to use these services is changing patients' relationships with health, illness and their own bodies.

The backdrop to these changes in healthcare and patient experiences was the emergence of a Bhutanese nation-state, including but not limited to more than a century of monarchical rule (1907 to 2008) and the more recent transition to a democratically elected government starting in 2008. Sonam Kinga's (2009) *Polity, Kingship and Democracy: A Biography of the Bhutanese State* offers one of the best narratives for the state's development. It describes in detail the consolidation and then de-centralization of state power by the succession of Bhutan's five kings. They were responsible for many of the state-building endeavours, such as taxation reform (2009: 255–57), the founding of a National Assembly and legislation (2009: 226–42; see also Whitecross 2004), the creation of a standing army (2009: 242–45), the formation of government ministries and institutions (2009: 283–87), the systematization of five-year development plans and the introduction of GNH as a replacement for GDP to guide development. Kinga argues that the 2008 abdication of King Jigme Khesar Namgyel Wangchuck and subsequent transition to a parliamentary democracy was a slow and intentional process of de-centralization of power away from a single monarch, 'empowering local communities in self-governance' (2009: 273) as well as the newly formed democratic government (2009: 320–23). Through the past century, Bhutan has entered a new era in which people have emerged as citizens of the Bhutan state. These citizens have been presented with a growing number of state services, authorized, operated and provided by state institutions. The Ministry of Health and the provision of free healthcare services were two of the most visible signs of state development, offering new horizons to clinical care and survival possibilities. As a result, sick persons now have a two-option healthcare system to choose from.

The first major healthcare route available for patients is the biomedical[3] services offered nationwide by the Ministry of Health and its clinical hospitals, Basic Health Units (BHU) and outreach clinics. Also called 'modern', 'Western' or 'allopathic' medicine, these services are the only biomedical diagnosis and treatment options for ill persons, with private practices currently disallowed by the Royal Government of Bhutan. Therefore, the network of care offered in biomedical treatment centres is the single largest centralized and funded healing source in Bhutan, with the ministry reporting a total of 1,990,958 cases accessing its nationwide services in 2012 (MoHa 2013: 66). The largest biomedical hospital, the Jigme Dorji Wangchuk National Referral Hospital, is

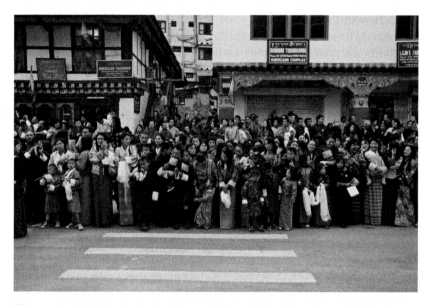

Illustration 0.2 Awaiting the King and Queen, *Thimphu.* On October 13, 2011, King Jigme Khesar Namgyel Wangchuck was married to Jetsun Pema, a twenty-one-year-old student. After the wedding ceremony in Punakha, the married couple returned to Thimphu and walked its streets, lined by throngs of celebrating onlookers. Celebrations continued for many weeks across Bhutan.

based in Thimphu, while the eastern regions of Bhutan are served by the second largest, Mongar Eastern Regional Referral Hospital.

The second option for sick persons is the traditional-medicine services offered within the Ministry of Health's institutionalized healthcare structure. As a part of an integrative two-option healthcare strategy started by the third king when he founded the Ministry of Health in the 1960s, these traditional services were developed alongside and complementary to the biomedical services, albeit with a much smaller budget and slower rate of growth. They are offered under the same roof as biomedical services in hospitals and BHUs, an infrastructural development that underpins the Ministry of Health's policies of medical integration. As a result, at hospital reception desks across Bhutan, visiting sick persons are offered the choice to see a traditional or biomedical doctor. In Thimphu, traditional medicine is offered in the stand-alone National Traditional Medicine Hospital (NTMH), which is also the service's training, administrative and clinical headquarters. Patient use of the traditional services has grown over the past decade, with 131,692 cases counted in 2011 reported by the National Traditional Medicine Hospital's nationwide clinics (MoH 2013a: 99).

The medicine offered in this traditional service is an iteration of *sowa rigpa* (*gso ba rig pa*), often translated as the 'art and science of Buddhist healing'.[4] This popular Buddhist practice has spread across the world, with many variants of private and nationalized clinics and practitioners using its methodology and cosmology, most notably in Tibet where it has received the common name, 'Tibetan medicine'.[5] Its most popular name in Bhutan was 'traditional medicine', known in Dzongkha as *nang pé men* (*nang pa'i sman*), where *nang pé* literally translates as 'Buddhist' and *men* as 'medicine'.

Along with the state-run biomedical and traditional institutionalized forms of care, people are seeking out a wide range of other healing sources, which I call 'alternative practices'. The practices in this third category are known in Bhutan as 'local' or 'traditional' (said in English, sometimes in the middle of Dzongkha sentences), or by specific practice names in Dzongkha, Sharshop or other Bhutanese languages.[6] Alternative practices may include shamanistic rituals, bone-setting, religious ceremonies, oracle use, spirit possession, dietary behaviours and familial care (among many others), all of which take specific forms given the socio-cultural contexts of the communities in which they are practiced. I call practitioners of these curative methods 'alternative healers'.

My use of the term 'alternative' here does not derive from its common use in the West to describe an amorphous range of 'new-age' practices. 'New-age' practices have a small presence in Bhutan, but they are not popular and were seldom referenced by patients, healers or healthcare staff. 'Alternative' rather points to an ethnographic distinction of 'local' practices from the state institutions of healthcare that take a dominant and powerful position in the politics, ethics, and patient narratives of modern-day healthcare in Bhutan. This division of institutional from non-institutional was recognized by my informants in the language they used to discuss alternative practices. The terms 'local' and 'traditional' were very much set against the institutional practices. Therefore my use of the term 'alternative' was intentionally selected to tease out this ethnographic occurrence of 'otherness' embedded in practice identities. However, most of the alternative practices engaged by Bhutanese healthcare-seekers do show similarity to those from other Himalayan societies as described in an extensive literature, by Samuel (1993) or Diemberger (2005) for example, the spirit mediums called *pawo* (*dpa' bo*) and *pamo* (*dpa' mo*),[7] male and female, respectively. While regional cross-referencing is both possible and necessary for an analysis of these alternative practices, some of them also appear to be unique to Bhutan, for example the *ja né* (*rgya nad*) healers discussed in chapter 4. In the discussion of alternative practices, I will draw upon sources that describe this regional similitude while also offering clear definition to those practices, or parts of practices, that appear to be unique to the ethnographic context of my fieldsites.

Finally, it's important to note that a main distinguishing factor between alternative practices and those of biomedical and traditional services is that they are non-institutionalized and, in most cases, non-centralized, professionalized or standardized. Alternative healers treat patients in their homes and community spaces, often for a small remittance. They operate within communities, referred by word of mouth or from religious practitioners who forward ailing persons who have sought a religious solution to their illnesses. As will be fleshed out in the following chapters, the government and its institutions of healthcare are often in contention with these healers, deeming them to be either dangerous in their own right or distractions to patients from the timely and effective use of institutionalized biomedical or traditional treatment. Although the unmonitored and unauthorized use of these practitioners frustrates public health officials, they are very much a part of the healthcare-seeking narrative of the Bhutanese, who will often use them in conjunction with the institutionalized practices without notifying the biomedical or traditional doctors.

A Brief History of Healing Practices in Bhutan

To understand where these practices fit within contemporary ideas of health in Bhutan, it is necessary to look first at some of the epochal moments in Bhutan's history that still affect patients today. Before doing so, it's relevant to note that Bhutan's written histories are arrangements of past events that form particular historiographies, narrative versions that often have agency within present political, academic or institutional contexts. In writing such a brief introduction to Bhutan's history I have selected historiographic narratives that link directly to the birth of the Bhutanese state and contemporary healthcare practices. There are omitted events, persons and texts that could provide additional historical perspectives. For example, Bhutan was and still is inextricably tied to Tibet, China, India and other Himalayan regions; the histories of these countries and regions are incredibly vast, with libraries of texts offering overlapping details and perspectives that could add to a narrative of Bhutan's history. I have selected specific events that are important to understanding Bhutan's contemporary medical context, but there are always more sources, known and unknown, from which to draw different versions of history. I will attempt to show where I draw my historical sources from so that the particular agenda of my historiography – to explain how modern-day biomedical, traditional and alternative healthcare practices came to prominence – is clearly signposted in the vast historiographic landscape in which it resides.

Reliable sources for historical perspectives specifically relating to healthcare are scarce, yet a few good works help knit together an evolving narrative. Melgaard and Dorji (2012) have co-researched one of the most rounded accounts of the *Medical History of Bhutan*. Their work charts the first-century introduction of Buddhism to the Himalayan region, including the introduction of *sowa rigpa*. After these early periods, they trace the growth of 'modern' medicine (what I call biomedicine), including a detailed account of the growth of the Ministry of Health's institutionalized services. Such a historical narrative on the foundation of biomedicine in Bhutan helps to form a discursive continuum between eras of healthcare practice that were very different from one another. Alex McKay (2004 and 2007; McKay and Wangchuk 2005) offers another well-evidenced argument for the early beginnings of these biomedical practices through the presentation of medical and field reports from various British-Indian Medical Service officers that accompanied missions to Bhutan. He argues for the importance of the adopted English education model in offering a springboard for the sustained growth of biomedical knowledge amongst wider populations. These authors present the most comprehensive medical histories available of Bhutan, but other smaller texts offer additional insight. For example, Trashi (2010a and b) writes about 'The Chagpori Healers', the name given to the few healers who served the royal elite in the nineteenth and early twentieth century, trained in the Chagpori Medical College in Lhasa.[8] Such works published in Bhutanese newspapers and by health institutions are often the only sources of Bhutan's history of medicine and healing that are widely read by the country's patients and practitioners.

While these works attempt a medical history, many other authors, both from Bhutan and further afield, have discussed other subjects of Bhutanese history, such as the nation-state (Kinga 2009; Aris 1979, 1994b, 1986; Ardussi 2004, 2000, 1999; Dogra 1990; Ramphel 1999a–c; White 1984; White and Meyer 2005; Collister 1987; Rennie 1866; and Pain 2004), culture and development (Ura 1994; Ura and Kinga 2004; Pommaret and Ardussi 2007; Ardussi 2008; Hutt 1994; Aris 1994a; Aris et al. 1994), state institutions (Gallenkamp 2011), literature (Ardussi and Tobgay 2008), religion (Aris 1987) and linguistics (C. T. Dorji 1997; Driem et al. 1998; Bodt 2012). The sources of these histories remain scarce, and they have drawn heavily from records from British-Indian expeditions. However, new sources are emerging. C. T. Dorji in his compilation *Sources of Bhutanese History* provides a detailed bibliography of texts in alternative languages. Although he acknowledges the 'lack of definite historical material' (2004: 15), he lists alternative sources of historical knowledge including: Buddhist texts, religious and devotional literature, biographical epics and legends, archaeological evidence, state papers and official records (16). He calls for scholars to draw upon these types of knowledge sets and diversify sources of data. However, the limitation of texts in Dzongkha, Chökey and other regional languages, as well as problems of access to translation resources means that these alternative histories often escape studies based on the English archives in India (e.g. Collister 1987 and Kohli 1982). The most recent historiographical edition is Karma Phuntsho's (2013) seminal work *The History of Bhutan*, which offers a sweeping yet comprehensive view of the changing economics, geographies, politics, state and cultures of Bhutan, making use of some of these alternative sources.

Unfortunately, Phuntsho's work, like many of the others, explains little about the healing practices of the pre-1900s, offering only a cursory introduction to 'traditional medicine' (2013: 6–7). The reason for this omission is that there are hardly any written records concerning healthcare practices in Bhutan before the 1900s.[9] Only a few literary traces exist – for example, Phuntsho's description of the stealing of ancient Bhutanese king Sindharāja's *la* (*bla*), often translated as 'life force', and his subsequent illness. In the context of this king's mal-relationships with local spirits and the saving powers of Padmasambhava, the eighth-century transmitter of Vajrayāna Buddhism to Tibetan-Bhutan regions, Phuntsho notes how *la* is a 'pre-Buddhist concept of quasi-psychological property of life or constituent of a person in addition to the well-known psycho-somatic components' (2013: 94). From such 'pre-Buddhist' cosmological insights and their roles in the causation of illness, as well as the histories carved from the earlier cited works, we can make a few educated guesses about what health-care and health were like in pre-1900s Bhutan.

Melgaard and Dorji (2009) identify three broad historical phases of health-care in Bhutan, each marked by a significant event that was likely to have shaped patient-practice activities and relations. While broad, these are helpful in understanding what types of healing are practiced today and what notions of health are prevalent among patients. Again, there are many other versions of history involving the spread of Buddhism and other political entities in the Himalayan region that could be included here. It's important to note that Melgaard and Dorji's historical narrative is linked to the dominant Tibetan traditional periodization of history, emphasizing the spread of Buddhism (Tb: *nga dar*) during the imperial period and the later extension of Buddhism (Tb: *phyi dar*) after the ninth- and tenth-century civil war.

The first historic phase begins in 746 AD when Guru Padmasambhava and Tibetan king Trisong Deutsen (718 to 785 AD) introduced the religious practices of Buddhism to the regions and peoples of Tibet and the then-unnamed and non-unified Bhutan region.[10] As a part of this religious expansion in Tibet continued by a patronage of descendants, *sowa rigpa*, the central medical practice of Tibetan Buddhism, increased in popularity.[11] The Tibetan king's personal physician, Yuthog Yonten Gonpo, is often credited with writing the original text of *sowa rigpa*, the *gyü zhi* (Dz and Tb: *rgyud bzhi*, Bolsokhoeva 1993; translations include Rechung Rinpoche 1973 and Clifford 1984 among others), translating and implementing various medical treatises, and establishing Tibet's first traditional-medicine college, Tanadug, in Kongpo Menlung in southern Tibet (Micozzi 2013: 131; Tsarong 1981: 95). The placement of the first *sowa rigpa* institute in the southern Himalaya was no accident; the region offered a vast pharmacopeia of medicinal plants. The lands further south of Tibet were not yet called Bhutan. One of the names of this region was Lho Menjong (lho sman ljongs), 'The Southern Land of Medicinal Herbs', still used today. This region offered a wider variety of plants than some Tibetan areas given the range between its high and low altitudes (Phuntsho 2013: 6).

While the spread of Buddhism into Bhutan has been explored by many researchers (e.g. Phuntsho 2013 and Aris 1979), the introduction of *sowa rigpa* is less clear. Melgaard and Dorji assert that 'while Bhutan supplied raw materials for the manufacture of medicines, Tibet provided the institutions for Bhutanese to master the art of Tibetan medicine' (2012: 21). Without formal teaching institutions in the Bhutan region, physicians required a sponsor to study abroad. Those rare few that managed to travel to Tibet to study in institutes like Tanadug would most likely have returned to a personal physician position with their sponsor, probably a member of a ruling elite. The returning traditional physicians from Tibetan training were reserved for a small privileged section of Bhutanese society, inaccessible for most persons. Sick persons would have to find other ways of curing illness than relying on this growing system of healing. Therefore the pre-1900s practice of traditional medicine was closely tied to a patronage with Tibetan *sowa rigpa* institutes, a relationship and training that continued until Bhutan institutionalized its own training and clinical services later in the twentieth century, only then offering these traditional-medicine services to the wider populations.

Before the establishment of Buddhism, various other forms of culture and religion dictated daily political, agricultural and social life, as well as the healing activities of Bhutanese communities. The problem we have today is that we have very few reliable historical sources on this time. This absence is even more distinct when it comes to healthcare and healing practices. We simply do not have any data to accurately assess what people were doing to heal themselves before the seventeenth century.

Melgaard and Dorji problematically draw attention to a popular religion known as *bön* (Tb and Dz: *bon*) to explain these 'pre-Buddhist' cultural and religious activities, as well as a 'system of bön medicine' (2012: 10). Academics such as Samuel (1993) explain the risk of using Bön as such a definitive historiographic catchall: 'The tern Bön and its derivative Bönpo have been employed by many Tibetan and Western scholars to refer variously to all sorts of allegedly pre-Buddhist and non-Buddhist elements of Tibetan religion, often including the folk-religion cults of local deities. . . . Such usage conflates so many different things under the one label that serious analysis becomes impossible' (1993: 10–11).

Given the argument of Samuel (1993), Melgaard and Dorji's collapsing of pre- or non- Buddhist healing practice into a 'bön system' might not offer an analytically accurate historiography. Ultimately, we are left with so little written or oral evidence of medical practices at this time that we can only speculate about how people combatted illness. Nevertheless, from this complicated relationship with religious and practice identification we can conclude two points regarding healing practices from the eighth to the nineteenth century in Bhutan. First, both Tibetan medicine formally of the large medical institutions in Lhasa and southern Tibet and other forms of healing not specific to a particular institution or regional identity were most likely practiced by individual physicians and healers, with a high level of diversification between the methods and cosmologies driving their healing logic. Second, some of these practices and beliefs were different from the knowledge of *sowa rigpa*, known today in Bhutan as traditional medicine. What were some of these alternative beliefs and how do they influence contemporary patient narratives?

There are some useful principles to draw from Melgaard and Dorji's early history surrounding non-Buddhist practices to answer this question; for example, there was a strong belief that one had to protect oneself from malevolent sprits or omens that share their environments with local populations (2012: 10). In this life-world containing spirits, ghosts and magic, as well as the cosmologies that guide their power relations, protection could be achieved through mitigation techniques, typically defined by some type of exchange – for example, the performing of rituals and the offering of food or gifts. Phuntsho touched on one such example in his history of King Sindharāja and the stealing of his *la* (life force) by malevolent spirits angered by the king's desecration of his tutelary deities (2013: 94).[12] The loss of his *la* caused grave illness to beset the king, remedied only by a spiritual exchange performed by Padmasambhava. This grandiose story emphasizes the engagement with spiritual beings and life forces in the aid of a king's health. Unfortunately there are no stories documenting the causation and cure of a layperson's illness, requiring us to infer the use of such cosmology and practice in daily life.

It is important to note that these cosmologies and knowledges regarding spiritual beings and the healing practices deployed to mitigate their effects on health were not necessarily Buddhist practices, and may not fit into a Buddhist cosmology. Such divisions in religious and spiritual beliefs are present and exerting influence on today's patients who also learn the differences between a Buddhist deity and a village spirit, the latter often described in scholarship as a type of 'animistic' entity (e.g. Walcott 2011: 254). Such specialist knowledge dividing religious and animist cosmologies required the intervention of specific healers and religious practitioners who specified their practices to one or the other, or both. Collapsing animistic and Buddhist cosmologies is both analytically erroneous and dangerous for patients; seeking a Buddhist solution to a non-Buddhist-caused illness wouldn't cure the ailment, but it might aggravate it. Therefore, awareness of these cosmological differences is important as we trace the narratives of patients who move across philosophical discourses, as well as those of the traditional, biomedical and alternative practices.

While the division of these cosmologies must be recognized, the confluence of Buddhist and other religious or animistic beliefs from the eighth to the nineteenth century have also come to play an important role in contemporary conceptions of health. As Buddhism spread, its practices and teachings on health, illness, disease and death contested and ultimately merged with these alternative views. Over time these influences became intertwined so that at times they may be indistinguishable from one another. A fusion of animistic beliefs and Buddhism continues to emerge in the concepts of health and techniques to ameliorate suffering chosen by patients today. Many of these, including the use of different alternative healers, religious practitioners and spirit mediums, and their engagement with patients, spirits, ghosts, deities, ill luck, negative karma and fate will be explored in the coming chapters.

The next important phase in Melgaard and Dorji's historiography of medicine in Bhutan is marked by the founding of Bhutan's nation-state through the consolidation and centralization of political and religious power by Shabdrung (zhabs drung, 'at whose feet one submits') Ngawang Namgyal in 1616. For the first time in Bhutan's history, a single political entity was able to unite the regions of Bhutan under its leadership. This was achieved partly due to the consolidation and delineation of political and religious authority between two figures, the Druk Desi ('brug sde srid) and the Je Khenpo (rje mkhan po), respectively. While this period marks one of the most well-cited chapters of Bhutan's history, the birth of the nation-state (a historiography well-deployed by contemporary state-building projects; see Phuntsho 2013: xiii–xiv), it also marks the beginnings of formalizing and centralizing *sowa rigpa*. This is the period when a few traditional physicians either visited or moved permanently from Tibet to Bhutan to offer medications compounded from plants collected and prepared from the Himalayan plateau. As noted earlier, these physicians would have worked independently rather than as part of an institutional collective, with no formal traditional-medicine institutes forming until the mid-1900s. Thus the post-1960s institutionalized traditional medicine is very different to the offerings of *sowa rigpa*–trained physicians at this time. These doctors were predominantly available to the Shabdrung and his inner circle. Many rural Bhutanese at this time would not have had access to traditional physicians and would have used alternative practices in their local areas, again, something we know very little about due to lack of reliable sources.

The third phase begins with the coronation of Bhutan's first king, Ugyen Wangchuk in 1907. A succession of five monarchs saw the introduction and development of biomedical practices and education throughout the country. This was the first time a healthcare practice would cast itself nationwide, conglomerating doctors and health staff, some of them Bhutanese, under one administrative and clinical practice. Melgaard and Dorji note that 'while the influence of British colonial rule in India until 1947 had a major impact on the future development of biomedical medicine in Bhutan, it did not provide the same amount of financial support as in neighbouring areas such as Sikkim, Tibet and Nepal' (2013: 5). Bhutan was never colonized, but British India engaged with Bhutan through limited dialogues by various political missions both before and after 1907 (see Eden and Pemberton 1865, Rennie 1866, and Government of Great Britain 1908 for examples of these dialogues, albeit rather one-sided narratives given Bhutan records of these exchanges do not exist). Yet their interests were with Bhutan's external rather than internal affairs (Collister 1987). When Ugyen Wangchuk signed away Bhutan's foreign office into the hands of the British, the subsidy was 'a mere 50,000 rupees until 1910' (McKay 2007: 187). Even after several doublings of that amount due to Bhutan's accordance with British India's various demands, 'the cost of supporting the state administration and monasteries left little finance available for development projects' (187). Lack of financing and a general concern from the monarchs and

British political officers that Bhutanese 'culture' and 'traditions' would be eroded by contact with Western influences, especially medical missionaries who were the most available for prolonged stays in Bhutan, kept biomedical development in Bhutan at a slow pace.

Relative international isolation continued until the third king, Jigme Dorji Wangchuck (1929 to 1972), decided Bhutan's future rested upon a slow and responsible opening to the world. This began with simple internal changes such as officially ending feudalism and slavery[13] and encouraging technological advances like wheeled vehicles for agriculturalists who, up to this point, carried crops from villages to markets. These smaller developments are pitted against large-scale national infrastructure changes to government, institutions and national services. By the end of his reign, he was responsible for the foundation and growth of many of Bhutan's government ministries that ushered in a new 'modern' era, including the Ministry of Health in the 1960s as well as the Ministry of Foreign Affairs. This was also a period when a rudimentary road network started to grow, a trajectory of accessibility that is still ongoing today (Fischer and Tashi 2009). It was predominantly during Jigme Dorji Wangchuck's reign when biomedicine and traditional medicine, as formal institutions, really took root in the country, and 'services', including hospitals, clinics

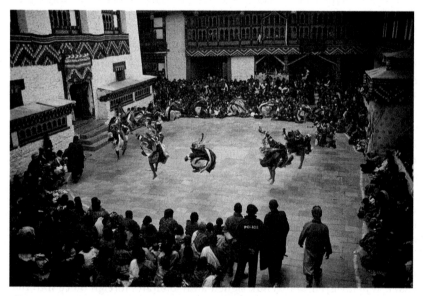

Illustration 0.3 Mongar Tsechu, *Mongar Dzong*. Crowds gather from all over the Mongar *dzongkhag* to come and watch or participate in the Mongar *tsechu*. Dancers leap into the air, pulling their feet all the way to their foreheads. Similar pictures are reproduced by the many tourists who attend these 'cultural' events, and they are often found in the large photographic books published on Bhutan.

and healthcare staff, were made available to the wider population of Bhutan. From this institutional growth, aided by foreign investment, expertise and medical schools, arose the government health services available to patients across Bhutan today.

From the mid-1950s to the early 2000s, Bhutan's slow and cautious approach to development kept many international influences at bay – for example, television was only introduced in 1999 (see Ura 1994; Aris and Hutt 1994; Ren 2007; Phuntsho 2004). However, with the 2008 abdication of the absolute monarch for the now ceremonial fifth king, Jigme Khesar Namgyel Wangchuck, a new era of democracy has brought an increasing rate of development and internal changes to the political, economic and social contexts of Bhutan.

This book is written against the backdrop of this rapid contemporary development and change, both in Thimphu and throughout the country.[14] Foreign influences have increased dramatically since the 1960s with the opening of trade, media, tourism, business and government channels with other countries. Increased wealth has also permitted material imports and the possibility of international travel for those lucky enough to afford it or those sent abroad on a government-sponsored trip. New influences are seen as part of a growing 'modernization', and materials, trends, objects, people, desires and bodies are often locally described as 'modern', highlighting their variance to a 'traditional' or 'old' identity. Sitting quietly in a Thimphu cafe observing the wealthy Bhutanese clientele as they sipped cappuccinos and discussed among friends, I overheard one woman ask a man sitting on an adjacent couch, 'Is that the iPad 2 you have?' The man replied, 'No, it's the Samsung Galaxy Tab.' To add to this observation, at a *tsechu* (*tshe bcu*), the colourful and expressionist dance seen as a vestige of 'traditional culture' held in the *Thimphu Dzong* (*rdzong*, ancient fortresses used for religious and state offices), one can often see iPads held high above the crowd, videotaping the performance. These are not tourists holding them but a growing number of wealthy middle-class Bhutanese living in Thimphu, who drive new cars, go out to restaurants, fly around the world or dream of doing so, frequent night clubs and engage in political debate. While the rest of the country admittedly may be far from affording such gadgetry due to the inequalities between urban and rural economies and development, the trend towards modernization is clear, with both urban and rural societies changing ever more rapidly.

In the midst of these changes, the Bhutanese have continued to fall ill and seek different healthcare opportunities. While the human constant of a fluctuating healthiness has remained, the ways in which illness is understood, experienced and treated has undergone massive changes, most of which occurred within the last sixty years. This book looks at some of these contemporary enactments of health, healthiness and healthcare as lived, suffered and experienced by many patients of modern day Bhutan.

What This Book Is About

From the cursory introduction to Bhutan, its contemporary plural healing scenario and its history, it is immediately apparent that ill persons and their families may call upon a diverse range of knowledge and practice to respond to suffering. Having spent some time following the narratives of ill persons in Bhutan, I discovered early on that most would use more than one type of practice, sometimes one after the other or simultaneously. Such an insight is no surprise to contemporary health practitioners in Bhutan, nor does it contradict historical records; since the dawn of institutionalized services, patients have oscillated between the two, as evidenced in a report from visiting international physicians Ward and Jackson (1965: 813) in 1965:

> While modern medicine is being practised increasingly in Bhutan, many of the older patients still consult local herbalists, who dispense powders and liquids extracted from plants. Sometimes the patients alternate between the ancient and modern worlds, hoping to get the best of both.

What results from this multi-practice use are complex healing narratives in which persons would encounter multiple forms of cures, conceptions of health and types of bodies in response to one or many illnesses and symptoms.

Beginning with this ethnographic insight of practice plurality, the first proposition of this book is to assert what a 'patient' is in relation to these cures (chapter 1). While the ethnographic nuances of this proposition will be fleshed out throughout this work, I start with a simple notion of what a patient is, and how one emerges from a social context, to identify the central subjects of my work: 'patients'. This is not a term always used locally, but, for the theoretical underpinning of the story I tell here, when a sick person places themselves in relation to a curative practice, they become a patient. A sick person is framed by the practices they engage and becomes a patient within the set of relations established and sustained between practice and patient. With diverse healthcare options available to the Bhutanese and their willingness to engage in them, sick persons were often becoming patients in relation to multiple practices, thus becoming different types of patients many times over. This praxis of a multiple 'relationality' between patients and various healing practices, and the not dissimilar work of Annemarie Mol on 'the body multiple' (2003), has suggested to me the term 'patient multiple'.

The second proposition is that patients are the nexus of decision-making in the healthcare-seeking process. In most cases, the agent of decision-making regarding which practice to use and when is the patient. This does not mean patients are independent or isolated agents; rather, many other social, economic and political factors and influences converge within a patient's decision-making process, feeding into the result. Family, friends, doctors, finances, geographies, topographies, advertising, public health education, healers, ethics, and many other actors could affect decision-making. Taking these influences into account, the patient is a nexus of decision-making between all three healthcare options. As we will see, the decision-making process for choosing which healthcare practice to use and when is a challenging and complex task for patients, especially when symptoms of illness have permeated the lives of these agents. The real-life deliberation over whether to seek traditional, biomedical or alternative practices caused an ethic of healthcare-seeking behaviour, to which proponents of different practices would attribute notions of 'appropriateness' (chapter 3). When should patients visit hospital, when should they visit their village *lama* (*bla ma*), when should they seek out the village healer or when should they take traditional medicines? These are all questions asked by patients and answered by a host of opinion holders. By looking at the patient as a nexus for such questions, I am able to fan outwards into the ethnographic networks to answer some of them, exploring both the personal and wider social influences that affect patient decision-making.

With these propositions guiding the methodology in the fieldwork, this book has two aims. The first is to offer the only ethnography of patient healthcare-seeking behaviour in Bhutan. It will show some of the factors that influenced the decisions of patients and the effect of these influences on their healthcare-seeking narratives. Put in the plural medical context introduced earlier, this ethnography explores the ways in which practice multiplicity was affecting patient's experiences of suffering and healing.

The second aim of the book is to argue for an understanding of the Bhutanese patient as socially multiple, defined by a praxis of multiplicity rather than an ontological theory of single 'patient-hood'. I will show that there is potential for the effective application of such a conception of a patient in health policy and operations. Rather than looking for the integration of practices, I turn to an institutional approach which recognizes and sensitively incorporates patient multiplicity to both attract patients to services, and deliver healthcare in ways that encourage effective, meaningful and safe care.

The current textual narratives concerning healthcare, its provision and patient activities in Bhutan have thus far omitted a detailed look at patient activities and the impact of practice plurality on their decision-making processes. Work focused on healthcare in Bhutan seldom explores patient crossover between practices, thus missing this potential application of patient multiplicity. The next section explains these textual narratives and where this book aims to add to the current literature on healthcare in Bhutan.

Textual Trajectories: Creating New Space for Patients in Context

Why research the ethnographic context of Bhutan's healthcare practices and argue for this theoretical conception of a patient? While many instances of medical pluralism have been documented around the world (see Cant and Sharma 1999, and Ernst 2002) or within the Himalayan region (Craig et al.

2010) by medical anthropologists as well as other disciplines, Bhutan's particular ethnographic context and healing socialities have yet to be noted in great detail. In particular, scholarship on medicine, health and illness in Tibetan societies has had a dramatic increase in attention over the past decade, with a growing number of Tibetan and foreign scholars writing on the general scope of health and healthcare through a variety of lenses, including Prost (2008) on Tibetan diasporas, Garrett (2008) on religion and embryology in Tibet, Adams et al. (2010) and Adams (2001) on science and religion, Schempf (2007) on mental health, Samuel and Cantwell (forthcoming) on long-life practices and Pordié (2012) on the social, political and identity dynamics of Tibetan medicine. All of these are primarily focused on 'Tibetan' medicine as practiced in Tibet, Nepal or India. Little to no work has been published on Bhutan, with its long practice of traditional medicine and medical pluralism being subsumed into 'Tibetology' and other neighbouring regions of study. This ethnography hopes to expand the ethnographic dimensions of Himalayan healing practices, offering Bhutan its own distinct yet connected place amongst this growing body of literature.

However, a textual lacuna is not reason enough to write about patient activities in Bhutan. More importantly, published research in this area can help healthcare providers in Bhutan better understand why patients are using different healing practices and concurrently how services might adapt to satisfy patient needs while maintaining effective care. This research is already being applied in healthcare reform, specifically aiding in the development of effective medical integration between biomedical and traditional state services, in coordination with the Ministry of Health.[15] Without understanding how patients are engaging with a consortium of practices, health administrators will struggle to bring effective care to a growing and demanding patient base.

Most patient narratives in the Bhutan-specific literature focus on either biomedical or alternative healing practices, with little published regarding patient activities within traditional medicine. The biomedical collection of reports are dominated by government or non-governmental-organization-funded projects interested in supporting or improving state services. Over the past six decades the Ministry of Health has hosted hundreds of biomedical research projects, exploring a vast array of health and disease patterns. I met many doctors and researchers, both national and foreign, during my stay who were engaging in biomedical research projects such as cross-border malaria (Gueye and Yangzom 2011) or nursing (Wangmo et al. 2007). These research activities and others within the biomedical practice are important to health staff for career advancement, but they also input important data into the ministry's policies and programmes. While such reports and the state-backed institutions that write them have noted the existence of other avenues of healthcare, surprisingly little has documented the crossover of patients between biomedical, traditional and alternative practices, often viewing such behaviour as detrimental to effective care. As one biomedical doctor put it, 'They [alternative healers] should be chased out! There is no use for them in healthcare in Bhutan today.'

Along with overlooking patient healthcare-seeking behaviour, there is a noted lack of research from the biomedical camp that engages with patient perspectives on health. Works that come close to describing patient perspectives, such as Alex McKay's chapter 'Bhutan: A Modern Development' (2007: 173–204), are upfront in noting the dearth of 'patient-based inquiries' (2007: 199). Melgaard and Tandi (2012) open their chapter entitled 'The Perception and Behaviour Related to Illness' in their extensive work *Medical History of Bhutan* by saying 'it is hard to find any information or researched literature about the perception and behaviour of individuals and communities when illness strikes them. Mostly, one has to rely on anecdotal evidence in various reports from travellers to Bhutan and on verbal memories of Bhutanese sources' (2012: 96). Two notable exceptions are Unni Wikan and Frederik Barth's (2011) anthropological study of Bhutanese children in the late 1980s, sponsored by UNICEF, which includes some details of patient attitudes to health, and a master's thesis by Amanda Duncan in 2008. While encouraging, the textual isolation of these pieces of social science research demonstrates the lack of interest from the biomedical camp to explore contemporary social changes and trends where patients are moving between multiples of practice and accompanying conceptions of health.

There is one centre of biomedical research in Bhutan that appears to be approaching patients' use of multiple medical practices, the Faculty of Nursing and Public Health (formally the Royal Institute of Health Sciences), the institution responsible for training nurses and health assistants who staff the numerous biomedical clinics throughout the country. Students are assigned research projects that directly engage issues concerning patient healthcare-seeking behaviour and the interface between the Ministry of Health's services and alternative healers. The topic is of paramount importance to these students given they will be working in rural communities, attempting to persuade patients into the BHUs without degrading community beliefs or practices. In a large darkened conference room I listened to over fifteen graduating senior health assistants present their research projects to the secretary of health, often detailing their attempts to convene a community around contemporary health issues such as domicile sanitation, sexual health or maternal care. Following a rigorous full-time course over two years, students clearly understood the government's emphasis on how to approach alternative practices: 'preserve culture and traditions, but ensure they don't hurt people.' This ethical stance was repeated to me numerous times by biomedical and traditional-medicine staff when considering patient use of alternative practices. These motivated students carry this knowledge and ethic into the field as they take on senior civil servant postings nationwide. Unfortunately not much of their diligent research leaves the conference room.

While patient use of traditional medicine has received less focus than its biomedical counterpart, other important areas of this professionalized medicine service have received growing attention with the National Institute of Traditional Medicine's (NITM, the official Royal University of Bhutan training institute for traditional doctors and health assistants, known also as the Faculty of Traditional Medicine) five-edition publication of the *Menjong Sorig Journal*, available online (NITM 2013). The articles both in Dzongkha and English cover a wide range of topics, including clinical therapies (Nidup 2009; T. Wangchuk 2009; Wangdi 2008), *sowa rigpa* diseases (Nidup 2010; D. Wangchuk 2010), raw-material collection (Tenzin 2008; P. Wangchuk 2008, 2009, 2010) and institutional structure (D. Wangchuk 2008). The latest edition extends the scope of the journal and the entire institution of traditional medicine with an article entitled 'Study of the Efficacy of Hot Compression', demonstrating a new and impactful focus on efficacy-related research. Arising from this journal is the only patient healthcare-seeking behaviour study conducted by Namgay Lhamo, a lecturer at the Faculty of Traditional Medicine, entitled 'Health-Seeking Behaviour Related to Sowa Rigpa in Bhutan' (Lhamo 2011; other versions include Lhamo and Nebel 2011 and Lhamo 2010). This study included a qualitative and quantitative appraisal of the 'awareness, treatment-seeking practices and level of trust and satisfaction' of patients (Lhamo 2011: 5) across six *dzong-khags* (*rjong khag*, administrative and judicial districts similar to counties). This is the first study of its kind, and it helped to identify and assert with academic rigour that

> the knowledge and awareness of Bhutanese people on sowa rigpa in general is quite good. However, there are variations among people with different social and educational backgrounds. People from urban and educated backgrounds showed evidence of better knowledge as compared to those from rural and uneducated groups.
>
> This study also noted sowa rigpa is quite popular not only among the ageing population of the country but also among the younger ones. This is because a significant number of people seek treatment from sowa rigpa and they were found to be satisfied and happy with the services received from it. Although people think that sowa rigpa medicines are effective and helpful to them, they still indicated the lack of complete trust and confidence on it for their healthcare. This is due to the fact that sowa rigpa still has to go a long way in meeting the overall health needs of the patients. Lack of modern equipment for surgery, emergency and diagnosis of internal ailments were the major concerns people expressed when discussing about its limitations. (2011: 35)

While there is still much work to do in understanding patient use of traditional services, this preliminary study serves as a fantastic springboard. One area for further research includes a requirement for greater locational specificity, given that access to services varies depending on patient location. There is also a need to study long-term service use and patient crossover between traditional and biomedical services. More ethnographic research would yield such results.

Patient use of biomedical and traditional institutionalized healthcare services has therefore received some attention. On the other side of the healthcare coin, an increasing number of articles and reports focuses on alternative non-institutionalized practices: for example, shamanic rituals, *pawo* and *pamo*, or *lama*-led rituals. Academics such as Francoise Pommaret (2009), Mona Schrempf (2015a–c), John Ardussi (Ardussi and Pommaret 2007) Tandin Dorji (2002, 2004 and 2007), Kunzang Choden (2008), Toni Huber (2013 and 2014) and Karma Pedey (2005) have done particularly extensive work to these ends, although the ethnographic context is still widely unstudied. Chapter 4 offers a closer look at these works and the practices they encompass. Alternative practices are evidently featured in academic literature focusing on 'cultural studies' but not in the literature produced by medical institutions such as the Ministry of Health.

The impetus for past research has generally fallen into two camps: the state service providers and those pursuing 'cultural studies'. The former seldom deal adequately with alternative practices, the latter rarely have access to biomedical and traditional services. Lost in the divide are the complexities of how patients move between practices and how this movement affects patient experiences of illness and healing. None of the work mentioned above explores patient cross-over amongst any of the three forms of healthcare, and thus it fails to address the full scope of a Bhutanese patient's healing narrative and their journey through a practice-plural healthcare world.

Many reasons for the division are found within the literature produced by cultural studies academics and state service providers. International research access in Bhutan is extremely limited, with government organizations tightly controlling the authorization and support of any research project. While this has protected the country from a host of corruptive or unproductive research projects, as well as allowing national researchers to thrive (see e.g. the *Journal of Bhutan Studies*, Centre for Bhutan Studies, CBS 2013 and the *Menjong Sorig Journal*, NITM 2013), government-authorized research often finds favour with the current agendas of the hosting institution. Critical research struggles to gain traction, as it does in any institutionally dominated context. In the specific area of healthcare-seeking behaviour, the far-reaching efforts by the health institutions of Bhutan to educate and persuade patients to use state practices (both traditional and biomedical) has meant that there has been little room for research into the myriad of alternative practices and the ways in which patients use them in tandem with the privileged state services. Emphasis is continually placed on the use of state services. Meanwhile, research inquiries into alternative practices are funnelled through an institution with a more a 'traditional culture' mandate. Research in such categories can struggle to make waves in policy and operations.[16] Thus for researchers wishing to trace patient narratives that bring both patient and researcher into hospital wards and then into the houses of alternative healers, opportunity is hard to come by. Access is typically granted for one or the other. This point of divergence is exactly where my ethnography sits. With access to biomedical hospitals, traditional-medicine units and alternative healers, as well as the everyday life of patients, I was able to follow the multi-practice narratives that characterize healthcare-seeking behaviour in Bhutan. The following section discusses how I structured this access in fieldwork methodology.

Methodology of Fieldwork in the Context of Two Fieldsites

The fieldwork spanned a two-year period and was composed of preparatory negotiations, a reconnaissance trip, remote research with institutional collaborators, a six-month ethics review process, a yearlong stay in Bhutan and ongoing contact with institutions and patients. Initial contact was made with Bhutan's Ministry of Health in March 2010, and the year of onsite fieldwork was conducted between April 2011 and May 2012. This fieldwork also fits into the wider span of my research experiences, including six months in 2006 conducting fieldwork in the Traditional Medicine Hospital of Lhasa, Tibet, six months in 2007 studying urban shamanism in Lima, Peru, and a year in 2004 spent doing health-related social work in a rural Nepali village.

To put it bluntly, gaining research access to Bhutan was hard, and it was a combination of strategic marketing, a preliminary trip, good council and sheer luck that led to my invitation to conduct the research in collaboration with the Ministry of Health and the National Traditional Medicine Hospital. The restrictions and conditions to foreign researchers are well-known to those who approach institutions with research projects. The reluctance to allow researchers into the country has preempted potential damage by research oversaturation (a country famed as the Last Shangri-la that coined and implemented GNH is particularly at risk of over-popularity), while also capping the publishing rate, in comparison with Bhutan's neighbours. However, as the new democratic government continues to grow and allow power to filter down to its institutions, more foreigners are being invited to work, study and research in Bhutan. The acceptance of this research project was a product of growing interest and commitment to research projects in general. However, tight visa controls still resulted in unavoidable adjustments to methodology.

I visited Thimphu for two weeks in late July 2010 on a reconnaissance and introductory trip. This self-funded journey was made after the Ministry of Health accepted an initial proposal, and I intended to formalize arrangements while gaining current ethnographic information to refine the research project. This was a crucial trip that influenced early changes to the project. For example, an interest in 'medical integration' between biomedical and traditional practices was rejected by my Bhutanese research counterparts – rightly so because it wasn't a particularly important factor to patients or health staff. My research collaborators at the Ministry of Health and the National Traditional Medicine Hospital helped to establish that patient crossover between biomedical, traditional and alternative practices – the ultimate focus of my research – was contemporary, important and unstudied. This trip also facilitated meeting with the minister of health, ministry officials and those affiliated both administratively and academically with the research project. The outcome was that the minister accepted the project under strict yet reasonable guidelines, including the accreditation of the Research Ethics Board of Health, which I received in conjunction with following the Association of Social Anthropologists of the UK and the Commonwealth's 'Ethical Guidelines for Good Research Practice' (2010). Another strict guideline was the maximum stay of one year in the country, a relatively long time uncommon for research projects that have no added commitment to teach or work.[17]

Having gained access, learnt more about the on-the-ground context, and met many healthcare administrators, my methodological plan was to spend twelve months conducting ethnographic research with patients, doctors, healthcare staff, alternative healers and patients' families. Overall I interviewed over 400 patients (formal and informal interviewing) and over 150 healthcare staff and administrative officers. I sat in on over 600 consultations in both traditional and modern medicine, as well as many other treatment and clinical sessions, including surgeries. I held three focus groups, each over a two-day period, with health assistants who work in nationwide BHUs. I also interviewed eleven alternative healers, three of whom I worked with over consecutive months. Many of these research activities were done with a research counterpart, who changed depending on my location and fieldsites. However, I would often conduct interviews and observation alone. These activities were done in two fieldsites, Thimphu and Mongar. The change in location marked two distinct phases of my research, both with well-defined ethnographic focuses.

The first phase consisted of five months based in Thimphu (population approximately eighty thousand, NSB 2005: 9), Bhutan's capital and home of the Ministry of Health, National Traditional Medicine Hospital and the Jigme Dorji Wangchuck National Referral Hospital. This is the largest and most economically and politically dominant urban centre, with all major government, monastic, business and academic institutions, and international and national non-governmental organizations, headquartered around its city centre. The usual promises of 'big city opportunities' have brought rural populations flooding in (Chupein 2010: 9), with construction projects quickly expanding the city along the Thimphu Valley. Taxis and private cars whizz round its bustling streets lined by busy office workers, students, businesspersons, shoppers, tourists, monks, nuns and stray dogs. Thimphu's development in just the last five years has been staggering. Where only five years ago rice fields grew, now shopping malls, housing blocks and busy roads have transformed the environment from rural to urban. With these recent changes comes the feeling that Thimphu is on the tipping point of a massive social, economic and infrastructural transformation, one where new trajectories of urban development are no longer new, but the norm, and with that normalcy a new era of modern city life is born.

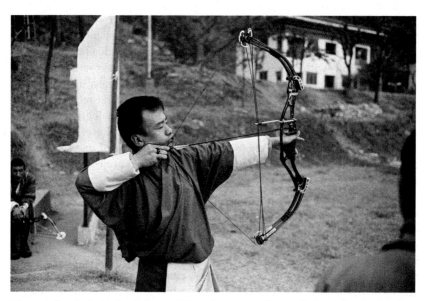

Illustration 0.4 Archer's Poise, *Thimphu.* An archer pulls back his bow, takes a deep breath and steadies his arm. The US-made carbon compound bow floats in front of him, ready to send the arrow whistling towards the target.

Amongst these familiar shapes of globalizing modernity are distinctive markers of 'Bhutanese-ness'. Many people still wear the national dress, a *gho* (*go*) for men and a *kira* (*dkyi ra*), or fashionable versions of it, for women. Admission to most official administrative and private offices is dependent upon this national dress, arguably helping to keep it in fashion. The nation's favourite dish, *ema datshi* (*e ma dar tshil*), a potently spicy mixture of melted cheese and chillies, still earns centre stage on dinner tables. The main attraction for Bhutan's recreational male is the city centre archery ground where arrows whistle through the air, propelled by expensive carbon compound-bows, echoing bygone battles with Tibetan invaders. Cinemas, *dzongs* and tourist hotels are filled with the 'cultural' sounds and movements of Bhutanese songs and dances drenched in the romanticization of epic love stories, the urbanite's bucolic village origins or religious and political antiquity. All of these things seemed to take up many waking hours for many of the people I worked with in Thimphu. If not in hospitals or clinics seeking or providing healthcare, my informants could often be found partaking in some part of these national rituals, either in real life or by the various media outlets. Within this urban setting I lived in private accommodation and divided my time between learning Dzongkha and conducting participant observation, interviews and discussions in the city hospitals with patients and health staff.

The introductory period to the Thimphu fieldsite and the Dzongkha language was successfully expedited and made easier by three factors, two of which had to do with my pre-fieldwork preparations.

First, I had a working knowledge of written and spoken Tibetan. Dzongkha (rdzong kha), the national language of Bhutan, shares much of its alphabet and grammar structure with Tibetan, and I was easily able to adapt my previous language skills to speak with patients, healers and doctors within the first two months of my stay with the help of one-on-one language lessons.[18] Although twenty-five other languages are commonly used in Bhutan (Ethnologue, ISO 639-3, 2013; Driem et al. 1998; C. T. Dorji 1997; Bodt 2012), there was no official avenue to learn them, and my time restrictions made it impractical to dedicate myself to learning popular languages such as Sharshop. Dzongkha, on the other hand, was spoken and understood by most of the people in my Thimphu and Mongar fieldsites and, given my previous training in Tibetan, was the fastest and most practical to learn. It should also be noted that English was the medium of education in all school curricula; therefore, English proficiency was relatively good, especially among younger populations. I argue that when researching an ethnography of Bhutan, English is a crucial working language, given how widely it is used, especially in hospital settings. Thus I used English as a secondary language of the study, when following an ethnographic trajectory involving the specific use of English or if Dzongkha or translation services were not available.

Second, my previous research for my BA degree involved six months of ethnographic fieldwork in the Lhasa Mentsi Kang (Tb: sman rtsis khang, 'traditional-medicine hospital') in Tibet, where I gained knowledge, insight and experience to both *sowa rigpa* in a clinical setting and to patient-focused ethnographic fieldwork methods. My familiarity with the *sowa rigpa* canon, its practical application in a hospital context, the medical language and theory, the institutional organization and the political tensions with biomedical institutional counterparts helped me to orient myself to this new yet similar ethnographic iteration in Thimphu. Also, I had worked with patients in Tibet, Peru and Nepal for over two years in other projects, and thus I was familiar with the sensitivities and tactics of interviewing and conducting participant observation with sick persons – an experience and exposure that I severely underappreciated the first time I worked with patients who were suffering.

Finally, although gaining access to Bhutan was incredibly difficult and took over a year and a half, once approved, with visa in hand, an endorsement from the minister of health, a collaborative working relationship with the National Traditional Medicine Hospital along with one of its traditional-medicine doctors as a research counterpart,[19] I was afforded ample access to health personnel, institutions and events. More importantly, the doctors, nurses, healers and patients I worked with were very encouraging and accepting of the research project and would often revel in the rare opportunity to meet, talk and work with a foreign researcher. I often described that the front door was like Fort

Knox, difficult to enter, but once inside, I was warmly welcome to visit any rooms I wanted and speak with whomever was present. I bought a car while in Thimphu that, combined with road permits processed by the National Traditional Medicine Hospital, permitted me to travel freely, again an extreme rarity in Bhutan. This relatively free access to people and places meant I could follow the ethnographic narratives on their own terms.

With access to the National Traditional Medicine Hospital and the Jigme Dorji Wangchuck National Referral Hospital, I spent my days observing treatments and diagnoses, talking with and interviewing patients and doctors and observing the use of medical resources and treatment options. If significant rapport was built with a patient – as happened with Pema, whose name is changed like all others in this book and who I discuss in chapter 1 – I would spend time in their social environments and follow their health narrative in greater ethnographic detail. I also interviewed many Ministry of Health officials across all administrative, educational, and clinical platforms. These officials were responsible for managing, providing and developing the public health services. They included the head of nursing in the Jigme Dorji Wangchuck National Referral Hospital, the nurses themselves and a trainer of nurses who was just completing her own PhD from an Australian university. I also held focus groups with select village health workers who routinely acted as bridges between rural populations and their local health clinics. As I was following patients, insights by those that worked in the gaps between homes and hospitals proved crucial to understanding the wider picture of patient migration.

Much of this work involved a 'bottom-up' approach to the collection of ethnographic material, locating answers to my research questions in the analysis of patient-based narratives. This is similar to the work of Lewis (2000) in his ethnographic narration of the illness and death of a Papua New Guinean man and to the work of Desjarlais (2003) in his biographic accounts of shamanic healers in Nepal. However, I attempt also to examine practices to move beyond narration and to infuse a critical analysis of sickness and healing into a body of regional literature that is heavily influenced by national politics. Throughout this work, I set new ethnographic material founded in patient experiences against historical accounts or government agendas. I do this not to criticize these narratives but to shed new light on the lives and activities of patients, so that institutions might more appropriately engage with the people they aim to help.

I did not limit my ethnography to patients who have particular diseases, such as many similar projects have done (see Mol 2003 on atherosclerosis and 2008 on diabetes, or Cohen 1998 on Alzheimer's). The study included all disease diagnoses used by patients, biomedical doctors, traditional physicians and alternative healers. This was a deliberate methodological approach because I was following patients who move between diseases, diagnoses and practices, sometimes for the same symptoms, such as a stomachache, or for multiple symptoms, such as an arthritic knee, a lost soul and a karmic imbalance. Following patients with a single classified disease is a good way of focusing a study and illuminating theoretical arguments: Mol's (2003) use of atherosclerosis to argue for her ontological notion of the 'body multiple' is a good case in point and will be discussed in chapter 1. This book is not concerned with making such philosophical claims, thus requiring a singular disease focus, but is rather interested in describing the life-worlds of patients in Bhutan and how subjects go about seeking care from multiple practices. It focuses on the movement between disease types and their corresponding networks of care, and how the plurality of cure, practice and body was affecting patients. Patients and their healthcare-seeking experiences were dynamic across a range of enactments, pain experiences, rationalizations and bodies, hence my choice to follow a multiplicity of diseases was reflected in the patient experience, rendering what I will go on to argue enacts the praxis of a 'patient multiple'.

The goal of this first stage of fieldwork in Thimphu was to gain a broad outline of national health services as they were used and propagated in the capital of Bhutan. The Ministry of Health and Thimphu hospitals were major policy and practice hubs in Bhutan. I intended to gather ethnographic data on these important sources of state healthcare narratives in order to understand how extensions of these powers were influencing patients in my second fieldsite in the Mongar Hospital as well as other national healthcare clinics.

For the second phase, consisting of six months, I was situated in and around the Eastern Regional Referral Hospital in Mongar town (population approximately 7,500, Office of the Census Commissioner, OCC 2005: 22) in the Mongar *dzongkhag*, which has a population of approximately thirty thousand, 80 percent of whom live in rural areas (OCC 2005: 22). The majority of these rural dwellers are subsistence agriculturalists living in the more remote areas of the district, some of which can now be accessed by farm or paved roads; however, transport services are limited, and walking to road heads is still common. Twenty-three BHUs and forty-six smaller outreach clinics provide basic bio-medical services. Two of these smaller health centres have a *menpa* (*sman pa*, traditional clinical assistant) that offers traditional-medicine check-ups, referrals and medication.

Mongar town is considered one of the largest and most influential urban centres in the east of Bhutan, although it is still dwarfed by Thimphu's prominence on the social and geographic landscapes. It is situated on the crest of a mountaintop, below which several valleys and their rivers conjoin in an epic display of rugged topography. It's known as a gateway urban centre between the eastern and central regions – all roads to Thimphu from the east went through Mongar, making it a major economic and agricultural centre. With this access, in the past decade, similar to Thimphu, Mongar has undergone a construction boom, extending its concrete Bhutanese multi-storey housing blocks down steep mountainsides. But unlike the capital, it retains more of its small-town feel, with agriculture still very much framing the surrounding landscapes and market trade.

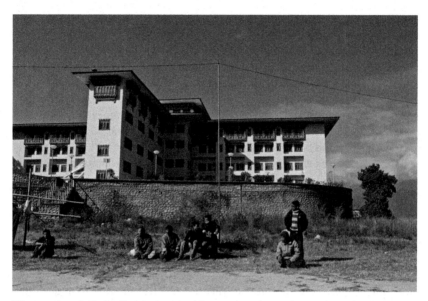

Illustration 0.5 An Eastern View of Mongar Hospital, *Mongar*. The five-story white wings of Mongar Hospital fan outwards from the central column. Each wing and floor houses a different ward or medical department.

The Eastern Regional Referral Hospital was completed in 2009, bringing newfound importance to Mongar. It serves as the primary state healthcare centre for the eastern regions, drawing in the remotest of inhabitants who sought the highest possible treatment levels on a national hierarchy of care, next to Thimphu. It offers biomedical services previously unavailable to eastern populations unless they travelled to the capital, such as surgeries, laboratory and pathology testing, endoscopy, obstetrics and gynaecology, radiography, specialized internal medicine, dialysis, and accident and emergency care. These services are supported by a growing number of biomedical doctors, nurses, administrative officers, ambulance drivers and hospital workers, most of whom live in nearby staff housing. I was provided with private hospital accommodation usually reserved for visiting international physicians.[20] The hospital also has the largest traditional-medicine unit, with two *drungtsho* (*drung 'tsho*, traditional physician) and two *menpa* on staff, as well as steam and bloodletting therapies. These two *drungtsho* and the traditional unit were my official hosts when in Mongar, as arranged by the National Traditional Medicine Hospital.

Along with these institutionalized healthcare options, the *dzongkhag* also hosts the second largest assortment of alternative healers in Bhutan, according to the Bhutanese newspaper *Kuensel* (Pelden 2012b) that reported over one hundred active practitioners. Although it's tempting to strike up a correlation between the number of alternative healers and the percentage of population living in rural areas, this would be falsely presumptuous, as alternative healers operate in both rural and urban populations. Thimphu is a good example of this where alternative healers thrive in the urban setting. Urban centres such as Mongar may offer a better location for such healers given their proximity to road networks, religious institutions and larger populations, all of which help to increase their caseload; for many alternative healers their practices are an important additional source of income and social capital. Clearly people in the Mongar *dzongkhag*, both rural and urban, have access to a large variety of alternative healers.

My initial meetings were centred on the Mongar Hospital. I first contacted the biomedical and traditional doctors and other administrative and medical staff to identify myself as a social researcher and not a medical practitioner (a firm and clear line I kept throughout fieldwork for ethical reasons – for example, I never wore a white coat, which would have given the impression I was a practising international doctor). When these relationships were well established, and agreed as appropriate, I started looking for patients to talk to.

Over the course of the fieldwork I engaged these informants in interviews, discussions and focus groups, and I observed diagnoses and treatments, including surgeries, consultations, bloodlettings, steam treatments, injections and general ward care. The aim was to collect patients' healing narratives, including the input and perspectives of doctors, nurses, healers and family members, thus creating a network of supporting narratives revolving around those of the patients. The institution of the hospital as well as the powers of the state healthcare system were important in the structure and ethnographic content of these patient narratives; I treat these state influences as narratives in and of themselves, therefore collecting biographies of the state and its health practices.

Through these relationships formed around the hospital, I also extended my informant base away from the hospital and into surrounding areas. This included accepting invitations to villages in rural areas, accompanying the *dzongkhag* ambulance, visiting BHUs or other hospitals and clinics, attending religious ceremonies, eating in the homes of patients and staff, participating in social events, travelling with hospital staff on outreach clinics to remote areas or restricted monasteries and meditation centres, visiting with alternative healers and spending time in garages fixing my car (dubbed 'The Tuna Can'). In total I visited ten different hospitals and ten BHUs, as well as a number of remote outreach clinics and healers' homes. Again, the focus of these social excursions was to add greater ethnographic detail to patient and state narratives, as they extended away from institutionalized services and into the socialities of everyday life in Mongar.

The data collected from these sites and ethnographic methods were recorded in a secure database designed and built from the ground up by myself, using Filemaker Pro. Creating a bespoke database solution for this project allowed me to record fieldnotes specific to the patient, practice and material narratives designed in the fieldwork methodology. I kept specific notes on events (including daily journalling), persons and materials, all of which were interconnected and cross-referenced through a confidential coding system. I also used audio recording and photography, with permission, to accurately capture interviews, discussions and observations. All photographs presented in the book are my own. Some photographs were taken at the time or place of events described; some were not and are illustrative of the ethnography.

Chapter Overviews

The book has five chapters and a conclusion.

Chapter 1 argues for the concept of a 'patient multiple', a subject category that I use throughout the work to better place patients in relationship to the many types of practices, healths and bodies they engage with during one or many illnesses. This theoretical claim is drawn from the following of a patient narrative, that of Pema, with whom I worked closely during my fieldwork and continued to do so through the writing period. I trace her interaction with biomedical, traditional and alternative healing practices as she attempted to cure two different health problems. In doing so I also introduce more thoroughly these healing practices, setting them up for further analysis in the following chapters.

The second chapter explores the traditional-medicine services and their effects on patients' experiences of suffering and healing. The first section looks at the use of the term 'traditional' and how it was used by informants. This terminology is important because it was used by patients and health staff to clearly delineate between practices, themes of segregation and inclusion that had meaningful effect on patient healthcare-seeking narratives. The next section looks at the organizational structure of these services, both in Thimphu and across a national network of clinical centres. By doing so I introduce the forms of institutionalization, nationalization and professionalization that are going on to affect what 'traditional medicine' is in Bhutan, as well as how it was enacting its patients. The chapter then explores how traditional-medicine patients are created within this institutional healthcare service. It takes a close look at medical records and consultations to show, in ethnographic detail, the interaction between practice and patient. The final section explores how the conjunction of the traditional institution and traditional patient creates new forms of ethics, bodies, and conceptions of health, as defined by the knowledge and practice of *sowa rigpa*. I argue that because traditional medicine is incorporated into a state healthcare project moving towards a rapid nationalization of services, what is beginning to happen is the formation of a new type of citizenship, one defined by a *sowa rigpa* body, health and practice. Patients' experiences of suffering and healing are then ultimately shaped and enacted by these new forms of *sowa rigpa* national identity, or what I call 'bio-traditional citizenship'.

The third chapter looks at the effects of practice plurality on the processes of patient decision-making. It looks at two specific ethnographic cases where healthcare decision-makers had to choose between practices, charting the influences and logics that persuaded certain healthcare-seeking behaviour. The first patient narrative is that of a newborn child who was failing to feed and as a result became dangerously dehydrated and jaundiced. The parents, Tshomo and Sonam, oscillated between visiting Mongar Hospital and conducting religious rituals. The second vignette is that of Dechen, a young girl with chronic arm pain, who was treated with religious rituals for three months before being taken to Mongar Hospital. These narratives reveal critical healthcare decision-making junctures, where the patients were at risk of death, and decisions between practices had to be made. Through the logic of care presented by the decision-makers as well as the staff of the Mongar Hospital and public health programming, we learn about an emerging ethics of 'appropriate healthcare-seeking behaviour' and how patients are implementing and navigating such ethical discourses.

The fourth chapter considers how alternative practices affect patient experiences of illness. It starts by looking at the contemporary world of alternative healers in Mongar and Bhutan at large, placing their practices and patient interactions in the context of specific political, social and economic networks that were in some ways defining their healing role. It then gets more specific, exploring a disease category, known as *ja né*, that was said to be treated by alternative healers. From my ethnographic data I identify three particular types of *ja né* and how each operates through a biomedical, traditional or alternative practice. The final section zooms in further to the *ja né* disease treated by alternative healers, whereby they practice sucking genital discharge from both male and female patients. I conclude by placing such practices back into the wider political and social contexts of healthcare in Bhutan, looking at some of the challenges facing such controversial healing methods. Ultimately, *ja né* and genital discharge sucking doesn't fit into a logic of care outlined by biomedical or traditional practices, yet it still holds meaningful agency for patients and healers, thus identifying a divergence in the way diseases are thought of and acted upon, again emphasizing the place of the 'patient multiple' in a modern-day Bhutan healthcare context.

The fifth chapter concerns the effects of medical materiality on patients. I first define medical materiality as things that adopt a healing identity and thus are active non-human subjects that exert influence on patients. The chapter then looks specifically at the increase in biomedical pharmaceutical availability over the past decade and the new networks of care these drugs have built up around patients. I look at the effect of these networks by examining what happened when they temporarily disappeared due to a nationwide drug shortage between 2010 and 2013. When Neyzang, a female heart-valve-replacement patient, dies, possibly due to inaccessibility to the drugs she had become dependent on, the ethics, supply and changing dependencies on such medical materiality are laid bare. I conclude by arguing that new horizons of what is clinically possible, as well as what is expected from the emerging healthcare services, has changed patient expectations of care. Rather than an unwanted pressure, such patient adaptation to and interest in medical materiality might pose novel opportunities for the Ministry of Health and its service providers; I argue that sensitive and wise advertising of medical materials might help to educate Bhutanese patients, result in more appropriate healthcare-seeking behaviour and ultimately reduce suffering.

The book concludes by first reasserting a call for patient multiplicity considering the ethnography presented in the five chapters. Second, it argues that the ways in which patient multiplicity is assembled, organized and managed by patients are what constitute healthcare decision-making processes. The ethnographic evidence shows that patients are very capable of understanding and layering the different modes of practice, health and body that arise from their narratives of healthcare-seeking. This organizing of the patient multiple constitutes a type of 'logic of care', a theory explained by Annemarie Mol (2008) that, if attended to, could offer new avenues of approach and support for patients by both institutional and non-institutional healthcare providers. By focusing service-provision efforts around the assembling processes of the patient multiple, we can better meet patients on their own terms, thus delivering more effective care.

Notes

1. The topic of hydroelectric power in Bhutan has received much attention due to its major role in the Bhutanese economy. Other sectors also play an important economic role, such as agriculture (Tshering 2009) and tourism (Singha 2013). However, the government has staked much of its future economic growth and stability on hydropower projects. For a recent assessment on hydropower's role in the Bhutanese economy see Ulmasova (2013).

2. As a side note to poverty statistics, there is a large gap in the poverty rates of urban and rural populations. Rural poverty rates went from 30.9 percent to 16.7 percent from 2007 to 2012, whereas the urban rate went from 1.7 percent to 1.8 percent. This detail to the statistics demonstrates two things: first, there is a wide income gap between rural and urban populations. Second, the dramatic drop in the rural poverty rate is informative to the growth in access and services to these rural areas over the last five years.

3. Readers unfamiliar with biomedicine as a cultural practice, once discussed extensively in medical anthropology, are encouraged to read Burri and Dumit (2007) and Lock and Gordon (1988) for an introduction to its epistemic, material and social implications. More recent summaries of anthropological approaches to biomedicine can be found in Lock and Nguyen 2010 and McDonald 2012 and 2015, for example.

4. A literal translation implies the term 'Buddhist.' Within Tibetan Buddhism, *sowa rigpa*, is one of ten 'Buddhist' sciences (Tb: *rig pa'i gnas bcu*).

5. Both academics and practitioners of *sowa rigpa* in Bhutan are aware of the practice's history with Tibet. Texts, lineages, institutions and training colleges for Tibetan medicine played a crucial part in establishing traditional practices in Bhutan. This is a complex relationship and historical narrative that is discussed at the beginning of this chapter.

6. Issues of terminology regarding alternative practices are explored more in chapter 1 and chapter 4.
7. The orthographic spelling and the phonetic transliteration of these terms are the same in Dzongkha and Tibetan.
8. The Chagpori Medical College was built in the seventeenth century by Desi Sangye Gyatso, the regent ruler of Tibet after the death of the Fifth Dalai Lama (Clifford 1994: 60). It is famed as the first medical school in Tibet, and it drew doctors from all over the Himalayan region to study Tibetan Buddhist Medicine. See Clifford 1994: 59–62 for more details of this Tibetan medical college.
9. Discussed through private e-mails with Karma Phuntsho, March 2013.
10. The introduction of Buddhism into this region occurred over centuries, drawing into it many important persons, events and texts, all of which are recognized but omitted here.
11. See Meyer 1981 for a comprehensive history of *sowa rigpa*'s development alongside Tibetan Buddhism.
12. Additional discussions on the subject of *la* have been written by T. Dorji (2004), Karmay (1998) and Gerke (2007)
13. Such monumental changes in political organization and social relations must be set against the political reconfiguration of Tibet in the 1950s, when the People's Republic of China asserted new Chinese presence and claim over Tibet (see e.g. Ura 2002). Bhutan recognized a potential invasion threat from the north and acted decisively to delegitimize any Chinese claims to Bhutan land. This included closer political relations with India and the British government, active engagement in the development of an autonomous nation-state and the change from practices such as feudalism that might legitimize an invasion by the Chinese who argued such practices as antiquated and requiring reform.
14. There are four notable publications that engage this 'modernization' trajectory. Rennie and Mason (2008) have compiled a host of contributions primarily from Bhutanese authors reflecting on these changes across a series of topics, including education (Yangka 2008), folklore (D. S. Wangchuk 2008), landscape (Gurung 2008) and culture (Choden 2008). Crins's book *Meeting the 'Other': Living in the Present* explores modern interpretations of gender and sustainability. The latter two works are by the prominent Bhutanese author Kunzang Choden (2013 and 2009), who is writing some of the most forward-thinking feminist fiction in Bhutan. These two books focus on the changing lives of woman in this contemporary development context of Bhutan.
15. At the end of my fieldwork (May 2012), I was invited to present a paper to the Ministry of Health, the National Traditional Medicine Hospital and the Faculty of Traditional Medicine on the topic of medical integration between biomedical and traditional services. This paper was presented in conjunction with a health consultant, Dr. Bjorn Melgaard, working on major healthcare reform in Bhutan. The paper and its integration policies are being worked into these health reform efforts that aim to achieve better communication and interaction between biomedical and traditional national healthcare services.
16. There are valuable and productive efforts to change this. A good example is the United National Solution Exchange Bhutan programme that offers a 'knowledge network to help development practitioners increase the effectiveness of their individual efforts, tapping into the collective knowledge and experience of practitioners across Bhutan' (United Nations 2013).
17. There are many ways to enter Bhutan to conduct research. One of the most popular ways for researchers that I met was to work for a government or Royal University of Bhutan (RUB) institution. Once present in the country, 'sideline' research projects were authorized, although work or teaching duties could take up much of the researcher's time. I had no work or teaching responsibilities and could therefore focus 100 percent of my time on the research project, again a rarity for someone given access to Bhutan for one year.

18. I would like to give thanks to my dedicated and trusted language teacher, Tenzin Jamtsho, of the Institute of Language and Culture Studies, RUB, who spent many hours helping me learn Dzongkha over the entire year of my fieldwork and beyond. His extensive knowledge of the language, as well as the social-cultural context of Bhutan, and his willingness to share it with me hastened and deepened my language-learning process. I would also like to thank the British Association for South Asian Studies for kindly providing a language-learning grant, without which I would not have been able to afford my valuable lessons with Tenzin.

19. Most foreign researchers working in Bhutan are required to team up with a Bhutanese research counterpart, usually from the hosting institution. I worked alongside a traditional physician from the National Traditional Medicine Hospital in Thimphu who was very helpful in all research planning and execution. Given he was a full-time doctor, seeing patients daily, he was limited in his availability to accompany me to many interviews and observations, other than those held in his office. Even with these limitations, he offered a great amount of knowledge and experience of traditional medicine and patient behaviours. I thank him for helping to introduce me so thoroughly to Bhutan, the National Traditional Medicine Hospital and the personal worlds of patients.

20. I'd like to thank the Mongar Hospital for providing me with this fantastic accommodation. They were extremely kind and accommodating to allow me to use it as my research base.

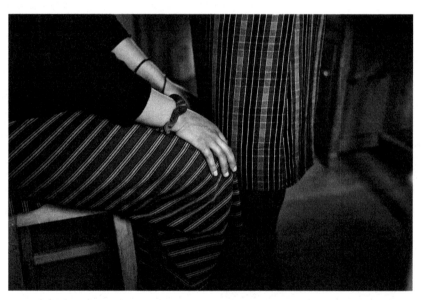

Illustration 1.1 Pema and a Drungtsho, *National Traditional Medicine Hospital.* Pema, a female patient, sits in front of a *drungtsho* to receive a nasal therapy treatment using herbal oils and facial massage.

1

The Patient Multiple
Cures, Healths and Bodies

Introducing a Bhutanese Patient

Early on in my ethnographic explorations of patient narratives in Bhutan I was struck by a problem. The 'patients' I worked with were using an array of healing practices, sometimes simultaneously, to cure their disparate health issues. The problem was that patients were so flexibly connected and constituted by multiple practices and knowledges that they fluidly changed subjective categories. Just when I thought I knew what a patient was and how they were being created, a new, contradictory or disjunctive subjectivity would emerge. Let me use Pema to illustrate the problem.

Pema and I worked together throughout my time in Bhutan, discussing the variations of her treatment history surrounding a painful and chronic nasal pain. She had visited the state biomedical hospitals, which had given her a diagnosis, medical records, medications and an operation. This single-track healing narrative augmented over time: two years later she arrived at the traditional medicine hospital with a bleeding nose and a resurgence of pain. She believed the biomedical doctors had failed as they hadn't dealt with the Buddhist aspects of the disease, and she hoped for a more fitting cure from these traditional doctors. Over the course of this one illness, Pema had already shifted her ideas of what the disease was, where it had come from and how it was to be cured.

Taking Pema's narrative complexity further, she then revealed she had another simultaneous pain in her stomach, however, this pain and causal disease was dissociated from her nasal issue. In her opinion, this disease had more to do with her astrological reading, or she called it her tsi (rtsis), and accompanying enviro-behavioural risks. I witnessed her bisect her body into two, both parts of which felt pain in different ways, explained through different understandings of health and curative practices.

How was I to deal with such multifarious patient subjectivities and ethnographic realities? To make matters worse, Pema was not a one-off case. In 2013, the Ministry of Health reported that its national healthcare centres treated just under two million cases, including returning and new patients in both traditional and biomedical medicine units (MoH 2013a: 66). In 1985 this number was below 350,000 (MoH 1986: 19), demonstrating a massive growth in the availability and use of national healthcare services. Meanwhile in February 2012, the popular Bhutanese newspaper *Kuensel* released an article quoting ministry figures that showed there were more alternative healers than all the doctors, nurses, health assistants and national traditional medicine staff nationwide, 1,683 to 1,593 respectively (Pelden 2012b). While these exact figures are contestable, they suggest a high demand for alternative healers as well as state healthcare services; across Bhutan, the sickly and those that act as decision-makers on their behalf are turning to many different healthcare practices to alleviate suffering.

This expansion and diversification of treatment routes in Bhutan parallels shifting ideas of health and healthiness. The arrival of new communication technologies, improved education and accessible health services in the past sixty years are just some of the factors influencing these changes. Not only are new modes of understanding and interpretation available – for example, with increased education and biomedical knowledge patients can now read and share their blood test results – but also new bodily interactions and modes of practice are easily accessible. Patients hook themselves up to dialysis machines, insert themselves into herbal steam baths or swallow new ranges of pharmaceuticals and herbal remedies. The new patient subjectivities emerging through shifts in both practice and knowledge are crucial in understanding healthcare-seeking behaviour.

The aim of this chapter is to argue for a theoretical conception of a 'patient' that will then play out through all following chapters, adding an important analytical position in understanding how people in Bhutan form coherent and effective responses to suffering in a diverse and rapidly changing medical scenario. I will draw from my ethnographic work with Pema, a nineteen-year-old woman with complicated and ongoing illnesses, as she 'becomes' and 'emerges' as a patient. I will describe how illnesses occurred in Pema and, through the course of their unfurling, through pain and understanding and in the company of different doctors, family members, healers and diagnoses, how she became not one patient but many patients, the 'patient multiple'. Through this narrative I will also introduce Bhutan's healthcare context, including the primary healthcare assemblages that go on to affect how, when, where and why patients seek out and participate in healing technologies, ethics, knowledge and practice.

The geographic contexts for the ethnography presented in this chapter, as well as the others, are the Thimphu and Mongar *dzongkhags*. However, the findings have implications and representation in many other areas of Bhutan. Latour's actor network theory explains how to 'transfer the global, the contextual, and the structural inside tiny loci[,] . . . allowing us to identify through which two-way circulations those loci could gain some relevance for others. [And secondly it allows us to] transform every site into the provisional endpoint of some other sites distributed in time and space[,] each site becom[ing] the result of the action at a distance of some other agency' (Latour 2005: 219). With this theory of network expansion, I defend the extrapolation of my ethnographic findings into wider communities and socialities in that Pema, as well as many other patients and doctors, have lived in other regions, towns or villages, some of which I visited while tracing healing narratives. With road networks and medical transport services increasing, patients now move across the country in search of a cure (see Tashi 2009). Additionally, both state and alternative health practices are relocating to and operating within communities in even the remotest of Bhutan's regions. While this chapter and many others will engage with geographic specificity and its affects on the ethnography, the two-way movements of agents – both human and nonhuman across a network, in this case the growing patterns in patient and health knowledge migration – permit a wider overview.

The chapter is broken into three sections, each introducing aspects of becoming, processes through which Pema becomes a 'patient multiple'.

The first section introduces the 'cure multiple', in which we learn about the variety of different health practices that Pema uses and relates to as strategies against suffering. I will argue that Pema uses multiple cures to meet her different health needs.

The next section explores the different conceptions of 'health' through which Pema assesses her own 'healthiness.' I will claim that Pema has multiple 'healths' that are afflicted by correlating diseases, which in turn require correlating cures.

The final section pertains to the role of the body in the process of becoming a patient, and how Pema has many bodies that both fall ill and ameliorate in different ways.

I conclude by describing how Pema retains a sense of coherency while living these multiples of cure, health and body. Furthermore, I argue that her use of multiple healing practices brings an agentive meaningfulness to her healing experiences.

While the triadic structure I deploy here suggests distinctive boundaries, these sections should not be analytically or ethnographically dissociated. They are all interrelated and interdependent, and sometimes they may be the same thing. Following Deleuze and Guattari's principle of connections and heterogeneity, 'any part of a rhizome can be connected to anything other, and must be' (Deleuze and Guattari 2004: 7). I treat the patient as a 'multiplicity' or 'rhizome', and thus adopt the theoretical idea that ethnographic subjects of enquiry are integrally connected to other subjects, or rather they are constituted by 'relations of exteriority'. For example, Pema's biomedical body part may detach itself from a bloodwork report and reattach itself to a religious modality of health. Her red blood cells are removed from the biomedical epistemology and mean something different in a karmically contingent cosmology.

My narration of Pema's illness is not limited to a chronological order, for it has been and continues to unfold over the course of one life that is still, at the time of writing, being lived. It began in the past, is occurring now and is being planned for in the future. It thus cascades itself across time, and I will treat it as such.

Furthermore in aid of arguing the muteness of chronology, my role as ethnographer must be considered. This story unfolded in my presence, as I sat with Pema during many consultations and treatments. It was revealed in interviews and informal discussions. Details were also communicated spasmodically, either during a phone call or a random meeting in the city. My learning of her story was not linear. Although my excessively zealous approach to interviewing attempted to sequentially obtain all the details of Pema's life at our first meeting, I quickly learned that systematically recording Pema's life in one interview was not feasible. In now writing Pema's healthcare narrative, I have found that sequencing her becoming a patient is also superfluous work, for the patient multiple does not lend itself to a linear or neatly packed chronology of events through time. The event of 'becoming' a patient has time, occurs in time, but is not dependent on chronological sequencing, or any sequencing for that matter; different orders and patterns of time are called into play when a particular chronology helps enact the patient of that moment. Therefore my method of relating Pema's story is purposely non-sequential so that our understanding of her will remain flexible and multidimensional, allowing me to introduce her as a 'patient multiple'.

Cure Multiple

Pema and I met in a small wood-walled room in the National Traditional Medicine Hospital in Thimphu ready to spend the next hour discussing her reasons for visiting the hospital. She agreed to talk with me after her consultation, as did all participants who joined the research project. She had visited the hospital because of a resurgence in chronic nasal pain and was starting a treatment course with a *drungtsho* (*drung 'thso*), the official name for a traditional physician in the traditional medicine institution. She was nineteen years old, a diligent and successful student from the Paro Valley, visiting her family and boyfriend in the capital city, although the boyfriend was a well-kept secret. She stood tall, nearly six feet in her high-heeled shoes, framed in a golden *kira* (*dkyi ra*), the female ankle-length national dress. My first questions searched for her beginning as a patient: When did her symptoms start? When did she first visit a hospital? When did she first 'emerge' as a patient? In her response, I found there was no 'beginning' in Pema's interpretation. She has always had people care for her using multiple forms of curative practice, and thus has been a patient as long as she can remember. However, one particular illness experience was singled out quickly as her most dramatic and memorable to date.

> PEMA: I was living with my parents in Paro, attending school. When I was twelve years old I was having headaches and fainting all the time. I was eating lots of medicine. Whenever I went to hospital they gave me paracetamol and vitamins. They said I

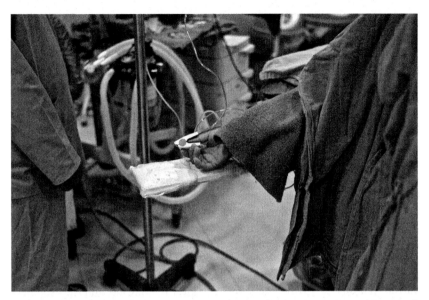

Illustration 1.2 Patient in Surgery; *Operation Theatre One, Mongar Hospital.*
A young female patient lies on an operating table.

was very weak and I should be eating vitamin C and taking lots of water and food so I wouldn't faint. I felt quite better with the paracetamol, but only for two to three days; after that again it comes. My uncle told me I should go to Thimphu and take an x-ray. I was thirteen . . . I went to the Thimphu hospital and took an x-ray. When the doctor saw my x-ray he told me that I had got a sinus problem and I had to do an operation.[1]

Pema's first narration tells the story of a one-track healing response. Pain occurred, and treatment was found. Through more interviewing, I learnt that the biomedical hospital had diagnosed Pema with acute sinusitis caused by a slight anatomical deformity in her ethmoidal sinuses, just between her eyes, where bone was blocking the sinus openings.[2] She underwent endoscopic surgery to remove small portions of bone to unblock the sinuses, followed by a heavy course of antibiotics to stop post-surgical infection.

If ethnography was easy and if all healing narratives were this simple we could stop at this sequence: pain → diagnosis → treatment → healed. However, I met Pema in the traditional hospital six years after her operation. Her chronic nasal pain was resurfacing, and this time she was visiting a different hospital, utilizing a different type of medicine. Not only that, she had formed new hypotheses for what the disease was and what part of her 'health' it was affecting, beyond just the symptomatic pain. This is just the beginning of a long and intertwined ethnographic account of Pema's illnesses and how she assembles a curative response. I came to learn that throughout adolescence Pema had participated in multiples of healing practices and would continue to do so over the year we spent talking together.

Pema, like all patients across Bhutan, has access to a plethora of healing practices. When sickness strikes she may choose from a range of responses and may often participate in multiple curative routes. She may assemble her healing trajectories from state-managed hospitals and health units, non-institutionalized healers, home remedies, corner-shop pharmacies, religious practices, dietary changes or familial care, to name but a few. As Bhutan continues to open its borders to trade and development opportunities, so increases the influx of foreign and domestic health-related materials and practices, the sole focus of chapter 5. Pema has resources that neither her parents nor grandparents had that increase her access to these new health solutions. She is highly educated, now studying at a top Bhutanese college, and has an outstanding literary competency. The bus she takes from Thimphu to her college uses newly constructed roads that are constantly expanding access to more remote regions. In her *kira* pocket she carries an ample supply of Bhutanese *ngultrum*[3] (*dngul kram*, the national currency abbreviated to *nu*) provided by her parents, who both work for the civil service, the biggest single employer nationwide, and thus she has disposable income for new medications and health products. With multiple cures arriving at her doorstep and the increasing means to access them, she regularly makes use of a diverse array of healing practices.

How can we conceptualize Pema's use of these multiple cures and understand what it means to be a 'patient' of these practices? Annemarie Mol has shown medical anthropology the importance of 'enactment', how 'medicine enacts the objects of its concern or treatment' (Mol 2003: 5). Following this theory, 'patients' emerge through the practices they enact. Without a practice, a patient is simply a sick person, a fleshy body deteriorating. This is more than just an abstract relation; it is a use of the body with technologies, people, epistemologies, knowledge and experience. A patient 'emerges' through the enacting of healing technology, ethics and regime and is thus relationally dependent upon the practices engaged with. With the diversity of practices available to Pema, she had to be categorically flexible, multiple, able to move between these relational enactments and be reborn within each practice. This is why it is so important to understand the various practices available to patients, as they will in turn define what we come to understand as the 'patient' and how that 'patient' understands themselves.

Categorizing healing practices can be difficult because of the diversity of practices that may be considered as healing, curative or preventive. The problem is both an ethnographic and a theoretical one. Ethnographically it can be challenging to distinguish a healing practice from something that may have nothing to do with 'health'. For example, would we consider T. Dorji's (2004) explanation of restoring a person's lost soul (*la tor, bla stor*), a practice common in Bhutan and detailed in chapter 4, as a healing or spirito-religious practice, or both? Would the practitioner who screams the name of the forlorn and bargains for the return of the 'life forces' (*sog, srog*, T. Dorji 2004: 598) consider it a health-related practice? There are even more mundane practices that an ethnographer might consider as a technology of healing: eating particular foods, circling a bus around a *chorten* at the top of a mountain pass or drinking *ara*[4] (*a rag*), home-distilled alcohol, hot and with butter and an egg. With the right lens, almost all human activities can be connected to concerns of health; it often depends on how far one is willing to go to connect the dots.

This ethnographic diversity makes it difficult to theoretically manage an assortment of practices. Clumping together or bisecting practices into categories or modalities risks either missing meaningful connections between them or conversely homogenizing variance. While this is a semantic concern dealt with by many medical and social anthropological theorists (Napolitano and Pratten 2007; Strathern and Stewart 2010, to name two of many), it also holds weight in the ethnographic sphere or, more importantly, in the illness experiences of Pema and my other informants; both dissimilarity and similitude of healing technologies have meaningful impact on their illnesses and how they thought about them. For example, as I spoke with Pema she was holding her traditional medicine patient record sheet, detailing her symptoms and diagnosis in Dzongkha. Her biomedical patient record also has similar data fields. However, the two state-run health systems don't share these records because they use different interpretations of disease and diagnosis; they are mutually unintelligible. Thus Pema has had to navigate the two separate yet informative diagnoses offered by these two hospitals. Two separate practices emerge through these similar yet disparate patient records, within which Pema must learn and interpret her illness. The question then stands: how do we talk about multiples of cures and practices without disenfranchising their ability to be multidimensional?

I navigate this problem by following Deleuze's theoretical language of 'assemblages', in which 'wholes' of things – for example, biomedicine as a practice and knowledge of healing – are characterized by relations of exteriority and not interiority (Deleuze 2004: 25). DeLanda sums up why the use of assemblages is valuable in describing ethnographic subjects such as biomedicine without pinning it down to a singular expression or entity: 'Relations of exteriority guarantee that assemblages may be taken apart while at the same time allowing that the interactions between parts may result in a true synthesis' (2006: 11). Biomedicine as an assemblage has a collectivized presence in patients' lives; for example, Pema enacts this medicine when she is injected with anaesthesia and then cut by a scalpel – this amalgamates a 'true synthesis', an ethnographic 'subject'. However, it also refuses the scalpel to be only equivalent or attached to biomedicine. When an alternative healer uses the same scalpel to cut into her skin, as described later in this chapter, the scalpel has moved across assemblages, multiplied, as too has Pema as the patient that interacts with that scalpel. By keeping groups or categories of practices as 'assemblages', they are both real for Pema and analytically transmutable.

Following Deleuze's language of assemblages, I begin by identifying three broad assemblages of healing practice from which Pema and other patients I worked with sought a cure: 'biomedicine', 'traditional medicine' and 'alternative practices.' Adding to this categorical approach is Byron Good's (1994) argument that anthropological understandings of biomedicine (or other categories of healing practice) 'consist not in proposing a series of propositions to which claims of truth or falsity can be attached, but rather in describing how medicine functions in various institutional settings such as in clinical or pedagogic encounters' (Das and Das 2006: 177). Taking this theory, I intend to look at 'assemblages' of healing practice as they are enacted by patients, doctors and healers in clinical and treatment settings. As Good notes, this does not include a clear delineation between practices regarding what is or what is not considered a part of its assemblage, but rather an identification of a particular practice trajectory as it occurs in the diagnosis, treatment and experiences of patients and practitioners, i.e. 'how it functions' in praxis terms. I will now follow Pema's narrative as she takes us through these assemblages in her search for cures.

Pema was young when her pain first started. She had a deep ache emanating from the top of her nose and between her eyes, a feeling of compression deep in the bone that no amount of rubbing or nose-blowing could relieve. She explained that as she sat in class she couldn't concentrate on what the teacher was saying; the pain blurred her focus as it spilt into headaches, giddiness and eventual fainting. After one painful night of little sleep, she awoke to find a small stream of blood trickling from her nose. She showed this acute sign of malady to her parents who swiftly took her to the Paro Hospital, close to their family home, where she began taking 'lots of medicines'. Eventually, this treatment route led to an operation theatre in Thimphu where she underwent a painful and traumatic surgery. What was this hospital and what regime of healing does it offer?

Pema's parents took her to what is the largest medical assemblage in terms of infrastructure, economy and patient caseload: what I call the 'biomedical' healthcare services offered by the state. Other names for this practice include 'modern' (*chi pé men, phyi pa'i sman*), 'Western' and 'allopathic' medicine, often used interchangeably by Pema, patients, health workers and medical publications. This institutionalized form of healthcare is administered by the Ministry of Health whose mandate is to 'provide free access to general and public health services in both biomedical and traditional medicines [and to] ensure access, equity, and quality health services' (MoH 2013b). These services have come a long way in attempting to meet this mandate; had Pema been born before 1960 she would have had very little if any access to biomedical services or any type of institutionalized healthcare practice. Pema is subsumed in the 2012 public results of this professionalized health service; she is one of the 94.4 percent of immunized children, she survived her birth and infancy in Paro Hospital marking the forty-seven per thousand child mortality rate, and having visited a hospital on presentation of her symptoms she falls into the 90 percent of Bhutan's population that has primary health coverage (MoH 2012a: 1).[5]

Although Pema used the Paro Hospital first, she could have accessed the biomedical services through the network of hospitals and BHUs spanning all the twenty *dzongkhags*.

While she received primary treatment and medications from the Paro Hospital, the x-ray and subsequent surgery required a larger and more sophisticated hospital, the Jigme Dorji Wangchuck National Referral Hospital in Thimphu. The capital city plays host to the administrative and clinical operation headquarters of the Ministry of Health, as well as various training facilities such as the Faculty of Nursing and Public Health, which is responsible for training nurses and health workers.

Pema, like many patients across Bhutan, was adept at understanding and utilizing this hierarchical network of care. In the search for better treatment, she requested a transfer to a bigger healthcare centre. I met one similar opportunistic elderly male patient suffering from chronic leg pain in Mongar Hospital, three days east of Thimphu by car. After he was picked up by ambulance from his local BHU (a service typically reserved for emergency cases), he was seen by a visiting North American orthopaedic surgeon, an international expert in his field, and a rare anomaly of professional excellence in this eastern region. Although the surgeon offered a compelling diagnosis and curative surgery by his own experienced hands the following day, the patient refused and requested a transfer to Thimphu. Longer queues, crowded operation theatres, high infection rates and an overstretched staff aside, the patient believed Thimphu to be the pinnacle of biomedical offerings.

Paro Valley has long been one of the most developed and accessible regions of Bhutan, playing host to the only international airport and the major tourist attraction of the mountainside monastery, Taksang (stag tshang, 'Tiger's Nest'). The infrastructural development of Pema's home valley meant that her access to biomedical services was direct and unencumbered. Patients in rural communities often face greater challenges to access similar services. Persons living in more remote areas may have to travel for multiple days on foot across rugged mountain or jungle terrain before reaching a BHU that may or may not have road access. Even if a road-head is nearby, some families cannot afford to lose a valuable labour hand during peak farm work months, or they may not be able to afford a taxi ride and will thus delay or forgo taking a sick person to a health centre.

Spiritual and religious beliefs also play a tangible role in accessibility and patient healthcare-seeking behaviour. Landscapes in Bhutan are filled with deities, spirits and ghosts, some malevolent, which have to be navigated to seek healthcare (Choden 2008). A nurse in the remote Lingshi area of northeastern Bhutan, which is four days walk from a road, told me that her BHU was built just above a small stream, and patients with open wounds would refuse to visit because malevolent water spirits (*lu, klu*) were known to enter bodies through

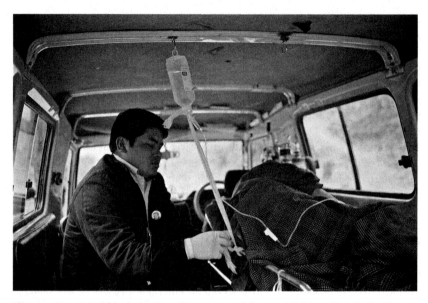

Illustration 1.3 Elderly Patient Transported from a BHU to Hospital; *Remote Village in Mongar Dzongkhag.* An elderly patient is transported from a remote village BHU to Mongar Hospital. In the ambulance the patient and equipment are firmly fastened to brace for the rough road back to hospital.

breaches of the skin. The Ministry of Health has long been aware of such issues and has deployed hundreds of 'village health workers', community members trained in basic biomedical healthcare, who aid patients' engagement with BHUs and hospitals through various methods of coercion, perhaps through financial means or simple persuasive reasoning. A growing ambulance service also aims to combat the issues surrounding road travel; however, limited vehicles that require tireless upkeep given the rugged road conditions are currently reserved for emergency cases only.[6] Patients suffering from chronic illness or those requiring check-up or follow-up appointments are more likely to eschew a visit to hospital. Doctors in Mongar Hospital often complained that patients from more remote areas would seldom return for important follow-up appointments and tests, often leading to further complications.

While Pema didn't have many of the complications facing rural-based patients, she did have her own set of challenges in seeking effective care. Thimphu's Jigme Dorji Wangchuck National Referral Hospital was overcrowded and understaffed. Queues for consultations were long with lines of patients filling the corridors. With approximately only one doctor per 10,500 patient cases (MoH 2012a: 63, 104), the demand was high and issues surrounding the under-supply of healthcare professionals were abundant: practitioner fatigue, rushed consultations, quality of treatment, misdiagnosis and high risk of infection

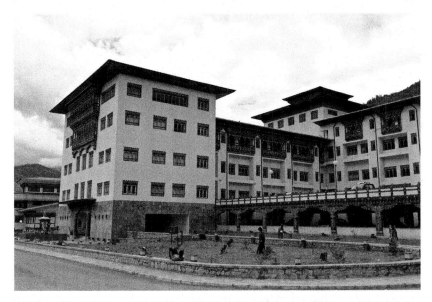

Illustration 1.4 Jigme Dorji Wangchuk National Referral Hospital; *Thimphu.* The photograph shows the main entrance to the new hospital building, completed in 1994. The original hospital building is still in use, completed in 1972, the front of which can be seen in the far left of the image.

were some of the challenges facing Pema and the administrators of the hospital (MoHa 2013: 10). She was aware of the difficulty in finding focused, timely and effective care from the biomedical services in the face of this overcrowding. Subsequently she, like so many other patients, worked hard to maintain familiar relationships with doctors or health workers. It was these relationships that secured her timely operation:

> PEMA: When it came time for my operation, the doctor told me they didn't have any beds. But later my father, he knows some doctors, he told them that I didn't have a bed and would not be admitted. But because my father requested, finally, they got one bed for me above the labour room, in the old building.

Similar to Pema understanding and manipulating the network of facilities, she and those in similar positions are increasingly learning to navigate the social networks of these biomedical healthcare providers. It took a doctor and me a good twenty minutes to walk the short distance between old and new Jigme Dorji Wangchuck National Referral Hospital buildings because patients and their families would accost him to chat, offer invitations or request personal mobile numbers. Friendship with a physician can offer direct lines of communication to service providers, which may help in finding quick solutions to accessibility and efficacy barriers.

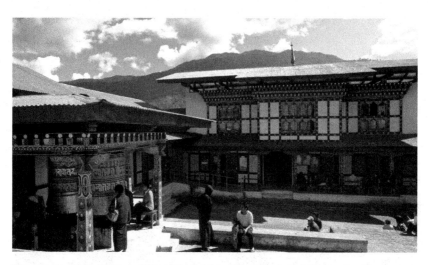

Illustration 1.5 National Traditional Medicine Hospital, *Thimphu*. The prayer wheels are stationed in the waiting area for the medicine dispensary. The rest of the hospital building extends to the right around the central courtyard, housing consultation and treatment rooms.

Having successfully procured a bed in the Jigme Dorji Wangchuck National Referral Hospital, Pema underwent traumatic and painful surgery in which her sinuses were cleared and widened. She recounted her fear of incurability or that her nose might have been completely cut off, as well as scenes of excessive bleeding, painful bandage removals and missed school exams. Although difficult to endure, both Pema and her parents were grateful for the biomedical services and the technology of healing they provided for free. Within a few months she had left hospital, returned to pass her examinations and felt much better.

However, two years later the pain and bleeding resurfaced. Frustrated, fearful and anxious about her collegiate studies, she revisited the biomedical hospital but was not satisfied with their offerings; thus, she decided she needed a different cure to her now identifiably chronic illness.

PEMA: It started bleeding again. The bleeding came for two weeks. Again I went to the hospital [biomedical], saying that I had done an operation and now it's bleeding. They put three machines into my nose and said that it had swollen up. My nose was swollen, and that's why I was bleeding. 'Are you sneezing?' they asked. I said, 'Yes, sometimes, when there's irritation. If there isn't any irritation, I don't have the bleeding.' They only gave me paracetamol and vitamin C. How are these going to help me? I told them again that I had done my operation and again I'm feeling unwell and bleeding. They told me to just get a nose spray, buy one and use it for two to three weeks. I did. But then I was not feeling well whenever I was taking the spray, I was feeling worse, and so I went to the Paro traditional hospital. They told me to come here [National Traditional Medicine Hospital] to do steaming and nasal therapy.

Having attempted to revisit the biomedical hospital and been dissatisfied with the outcome, Pema chose to use the second healing assemblage easily available to patients through a similar national network of clinics: 'traditional medicine' (*nang pé men, nang pa'i sman*). Arriving at Paro Hospital reception desk, she would have had the option to visit modern or traditional-medicine units. This time she chose traditional and was directed to a clinical room just off the main corridor. There she sat with the Paro *drungtsho* and explained her symptoms and history. The severity of her case prompted the *drungtsho* to refer her to the National Traditional Medicine Hospital in Thimphu, which offers a larger herbal pharmacopeia and range of therapies (see chapter 2).

It is important to understand the gravity of Pema's decision to use traditional medicine in the face of this serious development of her illness. When I first met her in the consultation room, she was holding a paper towel to her nose, stemming a bleed. She had just undergone a steam therapy and was discussing with the *drungtsho* her planned three months of treatment. She genuinely thought traditional medicine could be an effective response to her illness, trumping the biomedical services she had already tried. The government supports Pema's belief and is dedicated to using traditional medicine to improve national health concerns alongside its biomedical counterpart, creating a two-option medicine system. Pema also recognized that her engagement with the practice was emblematic in sustaining Bhutan's national 'traditions' and 'cultures', a subsidiary yet motivating force behind both patient and government support. Considerable financial investment in traditional medicine services demonstrate the commitment to these ends with the allocation of US$730,000 of the Ministry of Health's total 2009–10 budget of US$48 million to traditional hospital services and pharmaceutical production (MoH 2011e: 25).

As Pema inhaled the herbal steam and the *drungtsho* massaged her sinus cavities with herbal oil, she was engaging with an assembled healing practice known as *sowa rigpa*, translated as 'the Buddhist art and science of healing'. This practice dates back to the Buddha, who is said to have imparted vital medical knowledge, later written down in four medical tantras, the *gyü zhi*, by Yutog Yontan Gonpo between 708 and 833 AD. Over the centuries these texts have undergone various editions and expansions, changing the exact types of practices included in the *sowa rigpa* canon. Currently *sowa rigpa* is practiced worldwide, with some of the biggest teaching and clinical centres in Tibet, Nepal and India as well as Bhutan itself.

The tips of the *drungtsho*'s fingers rhythmically touched Pema's forehead in a circular pattern, and the pungent oil, made with thirty-two different herbs, seeped into her skin. Across the Himalayan plateau in Lhasa's Mentsi Kang (traditional hospital), another patient might have been undergoing a similar treatment, yet with an opposite rotation of the fingers; Pema was enacting one of many evolutions of this ancient practice. Many studies have shown that while the heritage and textual foundations of *sowa rigpa* are historically consistent, contemporary theory, practice and teaching varies across cultural, political, institutional, geographic, economic and historic lines. Janes (1995) offers one such cultural and historical analysis of *sowa rigpa*, specific to clinical transformations in Tibet alongside Chinese medical modernization. The work of Fernand Meyer (1981), Adams et al. (2010), Craig (2012), Samuel (2001), Pordié (2012), Saxer (2012) and Prost (2008), along with many others, continues to demonstrate the plurality and complexity of this practice as it spreads across social, political and medical landscapes. Resi Hofer's recent dissertation (2011) and book (2012) goes further in demonstrating the expanding territories of *sowa rigpa* by showing the importance of the subaltern histories of Tibetan medicine physicians who practice away from centralized institutions.

While Hofer's argument to de-centre ethnographic and historic sites for *sowa rigpa* from institutionalized settings applies well in her area of focus in Ngamring, Tibet, and possibly in other international regions where private practitioners flourish, the healing assemblage of traditional medicine that was treating Pema is firmly institutionalized, with growing standardization and professionalization defining how, when and where it is practiced. Like many other patients seeking cures, she accessed this practice through its state-run clinical institution and the affiliated pharmaceutical production unit and training college.

Pema's account of health-seeking has thus far focused on two institutionalized forms of healthcare made available by the Bhutanese state. These two medical assemblages are centralized, professionalized and nationalized into powerful healing resources for patients. However, Pema and patients like her often turn elsewhere for additional healing support that falls outside of the biomedical and traditional services' purview.

I call this large and summative third healing assemblage 'alternative practices.' Many of these practices might be called 'local' or 'traditional' (English) or by the specific practice names in Dzongkha or other Bhutanese languages. This incorporates the widest grouping of healing practices that have considerable variance between their technological, ethical, and social regimes. Practices include but are not limited to different kinds of shamanic healing rituals, oracle readings, astrology, bone setting, religious rituals, spirit possessions, herbal remedies, pharmaceutical and nutriceutical use, body manipulations, dietary changes, familial care and spirit offerings, all of which are leveraged by patients to treat illness.

One major identifying marker of this 'alternative practices' assemblage is its juxtaposition to the institutionalized and state-run practices, an important delineation that even Pema must learn to navigate if she wishes to use multiple practices. The biomedical and traditional medicine regimes are increasingly territorializing the discursive spaces of healing, the body and health. Patients are increasingly being framed within their knowledge, practice and administration, and in turn they are carving out specific types of healths, bodies and subjectivities – chapter 2 examines how traditional medicine was doing this. While public Ministry of Health initiatives do not reject all alternative practices, they are selective in spurning those they deem dangerous or unproductive. This has gradually led to a polarization between state-institution healing regimes and anything else that may be considered a healing practice.

In the illness experiences of Pema and many of the patients I worked with, this division between state and non-state healing assemblages was consequential, requiring honed techniques of navigation and intention. Pema often told me that she was 'scared' to tell a doctor what she had performed at home as a type of preliminary remedy, often preferring silence to a more descriptive narration, a common utterance from other patients. Furthermore, upon leaving hospital, Pema had many alternative healing plans, such as trips to an alternative healer, an astrologer, dietary changes and offerings to her village spirit, but these would be kept purposely private. This categorization of 'alternative practices' is not only for analytical ease but also to tease out the importance of this differentiated assemblage within the wider ethnographic context.

In my interview with Pema we began discussing some of these alternative practices she incorporates into her healing strategies. As a self-identified superstitious and religious person, Pema often visits alternative practitioners, both for her nasal pain and other health-related issues.

> PEMA: I go to the astrologers, *tsi pa* [*rtsis pa*], is how we say it. These are *lamas*. They will write my age and find out what's happening to me, what I should be doing.
> JONATHAN: How regularly do you do that?
> PEMA: I do it whenever I am getting sick. Most of the time I am getting sick so you know, I can't say in a year how much I do it.

Although private medical vendors are technically illegal in Bhutan, alternative healers offer an assortment of different strategies that often predate the arrival of both biomedical and traditional practices. The knowledges and practices used by these healers have been passed down through generations, and their services are still popular for even highly educated patients like Pema. The interchangeable terms 'local' and 'traditional' in regard to healers may be used to reference this wide variety of practitioners, although each healer may have a particular speciality and nomenclature, especially between languages and dialects. The Ministry of Health's 'Traditional Healers Training Guideline' (MoH 2011c) offers a preliminary list of these healers: persons who are embodied by spirits via ritual trance (*pawo* and *pamo*, T. Dorji 2007), spirit callers who return lost 'vital life-forces' (*la tor, bla tor*, T. Dorji 2004), female mediums (*nyel jor mo, rnal 'byora mo*), Buddhist treasure guardians (*terdag, gter bdag*), animistic healers using *bön* methods (*bön po, bon po*; Pommaret 2009; Schrempf 2007a; Samuel 1993), Buddhist horoscope readers and astrologers (*tsi pa, rtsis pa*), monks affiliated with a monastery (*lam* or *lama, blam*), lay practitioners or monks often not part of a monastic institution (*gomchen, sgom chen*; Tashi 2005), bonesetters, 'cuppers' or moxibustion healers, and burners by hot metal (*mé tsak, me tshag*).

Pema is not alone in her use of such healers. The National Statistics Bureau as a part of the Bhutan Living Standards Survey (2007: 25) estimates that in

2009–10 households collectively spent about US$1.5 million (*Nu* 80.885 million) on alternative practitioners and their medicines. While demand is evidently high, debate concerning their efficacy and future within Bhutan's growing network of state-centralized health services is ongoing in many facets of public and private life. Online forums popular in Bhutan[7] play host to vehement arguments regarding their healing and cultural utility.

Newspapers regularly publish stories that cast both negative and positive light on healer activities; see, for example, the *Bhutan Observer*'s 26 March 2011 article, '"Dangerous" Indigenous Healers Thrive despite Modern Hospitals' (Wangdi 2011). Discussions are filled with polarized opinions, stories of mystifying experiences, legality, rumours and intrigue, some of which are detailed in chapter 4. Within such discussions the exact practices, labels, categories and types of healers described and shared change repeatedly, making it difficult for an ethnographer, newspaper, Health Ministry or even Pema to pin down an exact practice. However, with the frequency of their use by patients, healers' interpretations of illness and their curative technologies play a vital role in the ways that patients conceive and experience illness and amelioration. Thus they remain de-centring yet informative agents within this ethnography of patient healing experiences.

Alternative healers are easy to identify in that they are typically one person offering a particular practice or ritual. Some of the other alternative practices that patients such as Pema engage with are harder to identify as they are often used as everyday technologies of the self. Yet, these more inconspicuous practices play an important role in her healing experiences.

Religion is one such example that plays an integral role in Pema's life, informing her healing experiences and curative practices. Buddhism has permeated (and will continue to do so) many of her major life events, such as childbirth, marriage, graduation, promotion, sickness and death. On an everyday scale, rituals such as early morning mantra and ceremonial offerings are performed in her household's altar room, with trips to monasteries and religiously significant sites taking up both professional and free time. Her school, like most in the national education system, insists on ten minutes of meditation at the beginning and end of the day. Visitation to a sacred site might render a handful of *ringpo*, herbal pills specially prepared by monasteries, said to have curative properties. Many of these religious practices that Pema engages in on a daily basis are thought to either assist in healing or maintain good health.

> JONATHAN: Did you do any *rim dro* while you were sick?
> PEMA: Yes, I did lots of *rim dro* and visited *lha khangs* [*lha khang*, temples].
> JONATHAN: Do you still do them now?
> PEMA: Yes, whenever I'm sick.

One of the most common religious rituals conducted across all regions of Bhutan is a *rim dro* (*rim gro*, *puja* in Sanskrit), in which monks are invited into a home, office or vehicle to perform Buddhist rites, sometimes lasting for many days. Pema and her family perform *rim dro* for major life events, to clear negative karma or to honour household deities. Pema also uses *rim dro* and other Buddhist rituals as a direct response to illness. Their curative qualities are well-known by other patients. I heard one story of a monk ushered to the bedside of a coma patient in the Jigme Dorji Wangchuck National Referral Hospital and permitted to perform a *rim dro*, albeit quietly. Within a day the patient awoke, perplexing doctors. In another story a family neglected to perform their annual *rim dro*. Shortly following this, a serious illness befell a family member. The recovery took place only after the ritual was performed, thus appeasing the household deities. Whether or not the *rim dro* caused these recoveries, illness often has a religious lilt to it because the persons who it affects are tied into the Buddhist cosmological universe, and the laws that govern this spiritual actuality must be acknowledged to live fully, healthily, in the world.

It's important to note that the term *rim dro* is a generic and widely used name for religious rituals that involve expressions of honour, worship and devotional attention to religious deities. There is a wide body of literature exploring the numerous different types of *rim dro* practiced in surrounding Asian communities and how these have changed over time. In Bhutan there are many different types of *rim dro* that match different deities, events, texts, Buddhist schools or life situations. A full explanation of this *rim dro*, its sub-variants and the other types practiced in Bhutan are past the scope of my argument here. I draw attention to them as a valued practice by Pema and many other patients as an alternative to biomedical and traditional healthcare services.

While Pema manages her relationships with the Buddhist universe, feeding deities their offerings, she too must pay close attention to what she feeds herself:

JONATHAN: So you have been taking the traditional medicine for one year?
PEMA: Yes. I was feeling better. But what I did then was . . . [she laughs and looks guilty]
JONATHAN: Oh no! What did you do!
PEMA: What I did was, the things I should be avoiding: I ate!

Like in so many communities around the world, the consumption of food and drink can change drastically in times of illness. Pema and her carers were actively changing elements of their diet to promote her healing or to remove polluting substances. In my contact with hundreds of Bhutanese patients I found that in almost all cases an illness event was accompanied by dietary changes. The most common of these was to stop the consumption of alcohol, spicy chillies, meat and occasionally dairy, eggs, tea or onions. The restriction or abstinence of chewing *doma* (*rdog ma*) – the national and 'natural' stimulant drug of choice made from betel nut, lime and a betel leaf – was also common. The staple of rice was seldom restricted, as were imported processed products, wheat-based foods, vegetables and water.

Pema was abstaining from meat, dairy and alcohol; however, at the time of her operation she also had to abstain from one of her favourite foods:

> PEMA: I had to eat for one month without chilli. I had never done this before. I never used to eat without chilli. Nowadays I eat two with each meal. But after the operation I was not allowed to eat chilli for one month. Without chilli I was not able to eat. I would beg, 'Please give me one chilli, please.' Without the chilli I couldn't feel any of the taste.

Such dietary responses to illness are often aimed at reducing the workload of the gut and stomach. Alcohol and chillies, one of the most popular combinations, is thought to induce and sustain stomach ulcers, a complaint of many patients, often but not limited to middle-aged men. The 'heat' of this irresistible cocktail is said to be difficult for the body to digest. Similarly, meat has an indigestible quality, especially pork with its oily fats. During illness, indigestibility can strain the body and take away from its own curative abilities.

There is also a religious element to dietary changes. Some readings of Tibetan Buddhist doctrine advise against the consumption of meat, as well as particular combinations of foods, an abstention that Pema worked hard to maintain. The traditional medicine hospital also provided Pema with dietary guidelines alongside its prescriptions, including the rejection of meat. *Sowa rigpa* has a long history of dietary theory and practice (Gyal 2006: 22), much of which correlates with wider religious and cultural ideas about food in Bhutan. When I asked my Bhutanese friends if they ate meat, many would bow their heads and quietly 'admit' that unfortunately yes, they did eat meat, it was often too tasty and too prevalent to not. This sheepish response is partly due to the religious belief that to be a 'good' Buddhist one must abstain from meat, which in turn promotes good health. Thus dietary change as a mode of cure is attached to many different aspects of Bhutanese life, religion and bodily functioning being but two examples.

Following the consumption of foods, Pema also navigated the growing number and types of medications:

> JONATHAN: Did you have knowledge about what traditional medicines were or what the other [biomedical] medicines were?
>
> PEMA: No [said earnestly]. They gave me the medicines and I just took them. I don't know. Now I feel as though I know some names of the medicines but when I did my operation and after my operation I did not feel as though I knew the names of the medicines.

It's not surprising that Pema didn't know the medicines she was taking when she had her operation. She was thirteen years old. But even as she became older and better educated it was challenging for her to keep track of the sharp rise in quantity and diversity of pharmaceuticals. Unlike her parents' in their youth, Pema had access to a large assortment of drugs through biomedical and traditional hospitals, as well as from privately owned pharmacies, alternative healers and religious institutions.

Street-level pharmacies are the only type of government-sanctioned private health vendor in Bhutan, with no other legal private practitioners or medical centres. While pharmacies do not provide consultations, they might offer Pema advice on the catalogue of drugs available to her, an inventory strictly enforced by the Drug Regulatory Authority (DRA). Bhutan is not like neighbouring countries where any drugs are available at a price, and at dubious quality levels. The Drug Regulatory Authority's regulation and policing of the importation of medication is extremely rigid to protect Pema from the potential flood of illegal or unsafe pharmaceuticals. The demand for new drugs is increasing, as is the demand for other types of non-biomedical medicines. One good example is the rise in 'nutriceuticals', the name the DRA uses for consumer drugs that walk the fine line between natural supplement and pharmaceutical. Bhutan's own traditional medicine practice is also starting to offer commercial herbal supplements and medicinal teas from its own *sowa rigpa* pharmacology. Drugs such as these and many other varieties are extremely new to the Bhutanese health market and offer a widening curative palette for Pema and other patients, a new form of medical materiality further explored in chapter 5.

A discussion of alternative practices wouldn't be complete without mention of familial care and the important role it played in Pema's visit to the biomedical hospital and her continuing chronic illness. While the doctors, nurses and health staff worked hard on her recovery ward, 'attendees' had an important role to play at her bedside, both in hospital and at home. In most hospital wards in Thimphu, Mongar and other regions, I observed that family members mainly fulfilled this role; however, a friend might occasionally accompany a patient.

> PEMA: My mother and father stayed with me [in hospital]. My aunties and relatives were bringing me food. My mother and father always stayed with me; if I had problems they would always be with me. Whenever I was having pain they didn't know what to do, but they would call the nurse. The nurse, because she is experienced, would do something, but I would feel happy when my parents helped me or stayed beside me. I felt relaxed and relieved.

In Pema's ward her family's efforts were crucial to her overall well-being. The limitation of staff availability meant that tasks such as feeding, toilet trips, cleaning the bed area, sourcing extra bedding and companionship were left up to her mother and father. While some wards may provide food services, many do not due to financial restrictions, leaving the sourcing of food and drink to an attending family member. Patients are typically allowed one person at their bedside throughout their stay in hospital, and the nursing staff will encourage the attending to stay throughout. Given that Pema was young at the time of her operation, her parents participated heavily in the communication between doctors and patient, relaying Pema's pain, discomfort, concern, fear, query or amelioration. For other patients and doctors that don't share a common language, a regular occurrence given the multilingual context of Bhutan and the growing patient migration around the network of clinics, the attending may act as primary communicator, who will then pass on the information or harbour it themselves to make decisions on behalf of the patient. This is especially true in cases where the patient has had little to no education, as more educated family members collect and action data provided by the doctors.

When Pema returned home, her family members took on the sole responsibility of care. Visits from biomedical or traditional doctors to her home didn't occur. In similar cases where a patient is homebound, alternative healers are more likely to visit a patient to perform a healing ritual or therapy, but they will stay only for the ritual and then leave. It's important to note that the home was a central location for Pema's pre- and postoperative healing experiences, with her familial care drawing upon a multitude of practices, medicines, healers, religions, foods, technologies, cosmologies and cultures. The diversity of Bhutan's healthcare context detailed in this section is condensed within this home environment, with many healthcare-seeking decisions made in the home. Critical decisions such as which healing method to use, when to visit a hospital, which medicines to take – all concerns of a new decision-making ethic engaged by public health programming detailed in chapter 3 – occur in Pema's home. Given this context of medical pluralism occurring in the familial hub, decisions are seldom individual; instead, they are formed from collective opinion and consideration from the family and surrounding community. When Pema's pain resurfaced, she went first to her mother in their family home.

> PEMA: I told my mother that I wasn't feeling well. I wasn't feeling well from going to the Thimphu hospital [biomedical]. I told her that I did my operation but still I wasn't feeling well. 'What's happening to me mother?' I asked her. She told me, 'Maybe you can go for treatment at the traditional medicine hospital where you can get another treatment.'

Following this conversation Pema changed her treatment route, with influence from her mother. This discussion was held in her Paro home, which was both a meeting point for multiple practices and the social setting for healthcare decision-making.

This section has presented a broad overview of just some of the sources of healing used by Pema and patients like her. The diversity of technologies, regimes and ethics of healing present Pema with a 'cure multiple', an array of practices that may in and of themselves or collectively alleviate suffering. Pema will use many of these cure multiples in response to illness, either simultaneously or in a compounding chronology. Like Pema, most patients that I worked with assembled complex responses to illness that involved more than one curative practice. However, as I will explain in the next section, not all practices treat the same illnesses, and not all illnesses are of the same 'health'. Thus an understanding of the cure multiple is not sufficient to explain what these practices mean for the patients that use them. We require also a comprehension of the different types of 'healths' to which cures are applied.

Health Multiple

Concepts of health – what it is, how it sustains and what types of intensities occur within it – are an important part of becoming a patient, a relationship that has long interested medical anthropology. Different ideas of what health is go on to shape the multiples of patients that may be found in Bhutan. Working with Pema, I came to understand over time that she did not have one stationary concept of health to which she ascribed her 'healthiness' but rather that she had multifarious 'healths' that were enacted through different practices, knowledges and phenomenological experiences of illness.

To understand Pema's conceptions of health, we must start with the most basic yet important observations from her discussion about the beginning of her illness and impending operation: bodily experiences of malady signal to Pema a problem with her health. 'Symptoms', defined as physical or mental features of a disease or illness, occur phenomenologically to Pema and in turn offer a barometer for her healthiness. She voices the occurrence of 'headaches', 'fainting', 'bleeding' and 'giddiness', symptoms defined as bodily patterns of illness experience, as markers of her healthiness. The operation and medicine worked to remove these corporeal expressions of illness, but 'again it comes', the headaches, the fainting, the bleeding, returning two years later. We may then conclude that phenomenological experiences of illness play a large role in how she understands her own healthiness.

This finding recurred in almost all the patients I spoke with in Bhutan. Bodies that break, rupture, suffer, bend, distort, open or bleed signal a reduction of healthiness. Like Pema's visit to hospital on presentation and persistence of her symptoms, these corporeal ruptures often motivate patients to seek healing practices. However, symptoms, either mental or physical, are not necessarily tied to a specific healing assemblage. For example, a stomachache does not necessarily turn a patient to the biomedical doctor. Rather, different symptoms call for different types of healing response. In this section, I will argue that these symptom and practice differentiations occur in part because Bhutanese patients have multiple 'healths' that require different curative approaches.

Pema's nasal illness and treatment choices offer a good example of a differentiation between a person's healths. Nasal pain led her to the biomedical hospital and an operation, decisions swayed heavily by her uncle, a military officer, and her parents. After the painful experience of surgery and a course of medication over one year, Pema recovered.

> PEMA: I had taken all those medicines from the referral hospital. And they told me that now I didn't need any more medicines because I was well. So they stopped the medicine. I was quite well for two years.

However, two years later her nose began to bleed in the early mornings. Pain resurfaced. Her body was again rupturing. This time she chose the traditional hospital, where I met her for the first time and conducted our preliminary interview. Pema was suffering from the same symptoms, but chose a different treatment route.

> PEMA: Later, when I was again having symptoms, I came here [traditional hospital].

One reason for Pema's choice to visit the traditional hospital has nothing to do with multiple healths but must be mentioned for transparency's sake. Most patients I met in the waiting rooms of the traditional medicine units around the country cite as a reason for visiting that 'modern medicine didn't work'. Pema expressed this concern when she revisited the hospital and was presented with a course of paracetamol and vitamin C, 'How are these going to help me?' she exclaimed. Traditional medicine offers a free and easily accessible auxiliary treatment route given its endorsement by the government. That said, availability alone is not the only reason why Pema chose to visit the traditional and not the biomedical hospital; after all, there are networks of referral and more than one doctor available within the biomedical services.

> PEMA: I was just thinking if I go to the other hospital [biomedical] they will give me the medicines which will help in one side but not in the other . . .

Another more complex reasoning for Pema's choice of traditional medicine is that her illness requires different curative tactics because of two different 'sides' of her health. Pema told me that her illness is with 'one side but not the other', referencing some division between two health states that require different healing practices. Pema was referring to something many *drungtsho* and patients would tell me repeatedly over the course of my fieldwork: that traditional medicine treats the 'root of the illness' while biomedicine treats only the symptoms, only the 'physical body.' This repeated statement highlights an ethical and spiritual hierarchy between two healths, one that is considered a base or foundational health rooted in religiosity, the other a more surface body-level health that biomedicine is effective in treating. This dualistic division explains why most patients would favour biomedical services when suffering from acute illnesses or symptoms, where 'acute' means symptoms connected only to this physical body. The best example of this is an accidental trauma like a cut, broken bone or burn. Most of the patients I interviewed would claim that biomedical services can cure these types of ailments better than any other because of its advanced technologies built for this physical body. Pema's nasal pain fell into this category, at least at first. When her pain resurfaced after biomedical treatment failed, it was thought that her illness was not only a body issue but also a deeper, karmically contingent health issue, thus requiring a practice that could approach her religious subjectivity. Buddhist cosmology and its comprehension of a person's connectivity within it play crucial roles here in informing this health subjectivity.

Marilyn Strathern, in her 1990 work *Gender of the Gift*, demonstrates how for Papuans the body was made up of many gendered parts that assemble to form a 'dividual.' She thus argues for the notion of an ontologically multiple world. Pulling this theoretical observation into Pema's example, and replacing 'body' with 'health' and 'gender' with 'healing knowledge', we can begin to understand how conceptions of health are constituted by healing knowledges. The concept and enactment of a person's health is assembled from multiple knowledges. In the case earlier, two healing knowledges are assembled by Pema, biomedical and traditional, each of which engenders her healthiness. Differing from Strathern however, I wish not to make an ontological argument here about multiplicity but rather one of praxis, or as Mol (2003: 5) might call it, 'enactment' multiplicity.

Unlike Strathern's dividual made up of dualistic gender categories, healths in Bhutan assemble from numerous combinations of knowledge and practice, not just a binary of biomedical and traditional. Earlier in this chapter I discussed multiples of cure, each of which enacts patients within different healing technologies. Each of these formative practices engages disparate health subjectivities. The best example of this would be the use of numerous types of alternative healers. There are different types of healers that deal with different health problems, not because the illness is itself different, but because the particular health subjectivity affected requires a diverse yet targeted response by the appropriate healer. Given that patients use multiples of cure simultaneously, it appears that healths and their corresponding cures cascade across illnesses and symptoms, forming a type of complex patient plateau upon which patient subjectivities are assembled through practice and knowledge.

Another interesting angle to approach multiple 'healths' is through Pema's understanding of 'disease' and how this relates to medical anthropology's wrestling of the term.

PEMA: My mother taught me that the traditional hospital will help cure your disease.

The term 'disease' as used in ethnography was disassembled and discarded by the medical anthropology of ten years ago. The discipline preferred to speak of 'illness' to sidestep biomedical territorialization, as seen to be encoded in the term 'disease'. The term 'illness' also posited the idea of perspectivism, meaning that the health object of inquiry could be seen from a multiplicity of angles, yet the object itself would be left alone, a Totality unknown, untouched. However, with the recent work of Mol (2003) among others, following Strathern's (1990) idea of 'dividual', there has been a new way of incorporating disease into medical anthropology's analysis of ethnography that moves beyond perspectivism and reclaims the object as it is, in multiple realities, thus emphasizing Strathern's call for multiple worlds. Mol argues that while the disenfranchising of the term 'disease' was necessary to deterritorialize it from biomedical coding, the takeoff into illness discourses has risked losing touch with the physicality and enactments that accompany illnesses. Furthermore it risks losing the agentive qualities of the term 'disease' as employed by informants. Mol urges the next wave of medical sociologists and anthropologists to re-examine disease as an important and agentive part of patient enactment. I follow Mol's call to re-imagine the term 'disease' as it exists for informants, both in and out of biomedical interpretations (see for example chapter 4 and the disease *ja né*). In Mol's understanding, 'this disease is being done' by Pema, it is enacted and 'depends on everything and everyone that is active while it is being practiced' (Mol 2003: 75).

In the traditional-medicine hospital Pema enacts a disease different from a biomedical interpretation, choosing instead a spiritual aetiology, namely a Buddhist one. The disease that requires traditional medicine's technologies is rooted in a Buddhist health, has pain symptoms and a physical body. Therefore this disease takes on all the physical manifestations that, say, a virus, cancer or infection might, yet it is housed in a different assemblage of practice and knowledge. Pema is highly educated and she understands biomedical biologies. Yet this does not disrupt the spiritual dimension to the disease; rather, it amplifies and informs it, and there is a religious physiology that is represented by her pained body. Thus disease becomes something beyond the biomedical assemblage, it detaches and reattaches to a Buddhist codification project but remains physically enacted in Pema's phenomenological experiences, encompassed by a mutually exclusive conception of health.

I have thus far attempted to contextualize Bhutan's healthcare context and argue for a conception of a 'patient' constituted by multiple cures and multiple healths. Pema's narrative has spanned across this medical landscape and patient subjectivities as she struggled to formulate an effective response to chronic nasal pain. Central to this ethnographic vignette is Pema's body, which has ruptured and repaired, and then ruptured again. If Pema's patient subjectivity is enacted through multiples of cure and health, what then becomes of this fleshy body? Does it multiply? If so, how? In the next section I will explain how Pema's body is also a multiple of sorts, a fleshy dividual through which she enacts her phenomenological experiences of pain and accompanying conceptions of health.

Body Multiple

This chapter has traced Pema's narrative of nasal pain and its treatment across two assemblages of cures and two conceptions of health. This section now takes an unexpected turn away from this sickness narrative into a surprisingly different aspect of Pema's illness experience, in which she bisects her body between pain experiences. This sudden and sharp textual shift mimics my own surprise at discovering how Pema had an entirely divergent illness to the one I had been following, a painful symptom and disease that was housed in a different health and body, requiring a different type of cure. It was only after this revelation that I started to fully appreciate the complexity of Pema as a 'patient multiple'.

I met with Pema a day later, after her visit to the traditional hospital and our interview. We happened to be in the same place to celebrate Buddha's birthday, at the Memorial Chorten, a large white monument known also as a *stupa*, in the centre of the city. Thimphu is big enough to feel lonely sometimes, but small enough to run into friends regularly. The *chorten* was busy, with all types of Thimphu dwellers circumnavigating the tall white *stupa*. The large courtyard was littered with picnickers, tourists, old diligent prayers and young Bhutanese students thumbing their mobiles, attempting to lure their crush to a public date. Successful young lovers intermittently held hands as they circled the *stupa*, a declaration of affection in a modern urban era, meshed together with religious continuity. Some may distain this flagrant showing of affection; others envy it as a youthful sign of social progress. It depends what side of the 'modern' versus 'tradition' war you are on.

Pema and I walked together discussing the religious significance of the day. Her knowledge of the festival was vast, well captured from fifteen years in the Bhutanese education system that promotes the learning and practice of Buddhist specificities. We paused at the back of the *stupa* and sat on the stone steps to watch the stream of karma-gaining bodies flood by. I asked her how her health had been since her visit to hospital. I realized that this was no longer a strictly research relationship, but one of friendship. The continuity of my inquiry from interview to informal discussion is a hallmark of ethnography, and I was about to find out why such lateral jaunts of methodology are so prized by ethnographers.

Pema told me that her nasal problem was not bothering her. She thought that the steam treatments, medication and massage therapy at the traditional hospital were having a positive effect, but it was still too early to tell. I asked more about the hospital and her reasons for visiting, but her attention was elsewhere. She hesitated for a moment and then quietly told me there was another problem that she didn't reveal to me during our interview yesterday in the hospital. Neither did she reveal it to the traditional *drungtsho* during her consultation nor the doctor in the biomedical hospital. She described a stomach pain deep in the base of her gut, a continual throb, a knot of pain, like a tight fist balled up and pressing sharp knuckles into the stomach wall as the wrist turns ever so slowly. She knew why she had this pain too – she had a diagnosis. Her *tsi*, a Buddhist horoscope reading often performed at childbirth, warned her of eating white-coloured food. At childbirth, a monk who told her mother, who in turn told Pema, that the composition of her body in combination with certain white foods might expose her to poisoning by malevolent spirits (see Choden 2008). Unfortunately it appeared that such a poison known as *dug* (*dug*) had been delivered.

Suddenly our previous day's discussion about food and traditional medicine shone in a different light.

> PEMA: You should ask the *drungtsho*, he'll tell you what foods you should be avoiding when you have a problem. For me he said that fish, pork, garlic and Datsi cheese is not good.

All these foods are white, and although the *drungtsho* had only recently warned her against them, it appears that they have been a concern of hers for some time. Perhaps she had reinterpreted the *drungtsho's* dietary suggestions to match her preexisting notions of her personal dangers surrounding white foods. Or maybe it was coincidental. Pema thought neither; instead, of course, the *drungtsho* told her to avoid these foods because her *tsi* and her *sowa rigpa* diagnosis are intrinsically linked. The multiplicity of healths and cures that this dietary advice pertains to are subsumed by a totalizing Buddhist understanding of food in relation to astrology. In this case, Pema was placing this curative technology of dietary abstention into one assemblage of medical knowledge.

However, this linkage of food and horoscopes was tenuous as Pema went on to dissociate this pain from her other symptoms. The eating of white food was not affecting her nasal pain because that disease was of a different health. Thus while the specifics of food might have spanned multiples of cures, being the same thing in different networks, the diseases were starkly different.

I asked if she had told any of the doctors or *drungtsho* about the stomach pain. She looked at me quizzically and rhetorically asked, 'Why would I? This is not something they can cure. It has nothing to do with them. I must visit a local *lama* to treat this problem. But I am nervous, because I don't like knives, and I'm afraid the cutting will hurt.'

She is discussing here a type of 'cutting and sucking' practice known as *trak jip kyap ni* (*khrag 'jib rkyab ni*, literally, to suck blood) or *ra jip kyap ni* (*rwa 'jib rkyab ni*, literally, to suck with a horn), administered by a Thimphu-based alternative healer. This practitioner is neither a biomedical health worker nor a *drungtsho* and does not have any affiliation with the Ministry of Health. He operates privately, from his home, like many others all over Bhutan. The healer may not be a religious figure, but many do claim affiliation with Buddhism or a monastic institution. This healer will take a sharp blade of some kind and make five bunches of six small incisions into Pema's stomach. The tip of the blade will score the top of her skin, splitting it to allow some light bleeding. He will then place the thick end of a hollow ram's horn around the cuts, and suck through the small hole on the other end. As the vacuum builds inside the horn, blood is suctioned from the incisions, as too is the poison in her stomach. This healing practice is accompanied by continuous mantras, incense burning and the presence of other protective religious materials. As I found out a few months later, this practice may have to be repeated three to five times, depending on the severity of the poisoning.

A week later I met Pema again; she had visited this healer and performed his treatment. She winced and sighed as she described the suspense and pain of being cut. She hated it and had cried throughout the ritual, holding the hand of a friend who had accompanied her. She was also distraught at having to return two more times, at the behest of the healer. Apparently her poisoning was severe and required further treatment. Yet her fear and squeamishness did not deter her from her healing mission; she would return to the healer the following week to rid herself of this poison.

The details of this practice, its variants and many others are described further in chapter 4. Here I want to focus on what is happening to Pema as a patient, as body multiple and as a pain experiencer.

I asked explicitly if her stomach pain had anything to do with her nasal bleeding and she said no. The two diseases (*né, nad*) were separate, and therefore there was no need to tell any of the doctors about this pain. The notion that the symptoms might be connected was nonsensical because they are of different healths and aetiologies, requiring different cures. What was unsaid but implied is the enactment of two bodies, each of which relate to multiple healths and multiple cures.

This phenomenological disassociation occurs within Pema's 'fleshy body'. Bleeding and stomach pain are fleshy processes that must be treated as such by Pema. For example, she chooses to cut into her body to relieve the stomach pain, a visceral, emotional and tangible therapy. Meanwhile her nasal pain requires medication that will reach deep into her fleshy body and realign her humoural balances. The enactment of these practices creates different bodies, body multiples. Pema treats these bodies through multiple healing practices, and does so with remarkable confidence. Emerging from these phenomenologically divergent pains are two bodies, bisected by Pema's enactment of practices, diseases and healths, as well as those agents, doctors and family that are active in doing these bodies. She treats her flesh as two bodies, requiring two different cures, occurring in two different health subjects. Thus her body is multiple.

At the root of this multiplication of Pema's bodies are the phenomenologies of pain and how they are experienced and comprehended bisectionally. This phenomenology is first foregrounded by her health multiples, arrays of sociocultural health knowledge that presuppose the experiences themselves. As Merleau-Ponty tells us, 'Now the sensation and images which are supposed to be the beginning and end of all knowledge never make their appearance anywhere other than within a horizon of meaning' (2002: 18). For Pema this horizon of meaning shifts depending on the types of pain and thus the particulars of diseases and their aetiologies, as well as the body plateau onto which these diseases cascade. This stomach pain and its corresponding disease (*né*) and diagnosis (poisoning, *dug*) was foregrounded in her religious concepts and her understandings of this body's cosmological makeup, as well as in relation to the socio-cultural healing practices that fit with these pains and diseases.

Following this foregrounding, Pema's body is then enacted in the phenomenological experiences themselves, sensations of stomach and nasal pain compartmentalized and dissociated. Pain, phenomena of experience, is simultaneously felt and interpreted. Pema's bodies emerge through these phenomena.

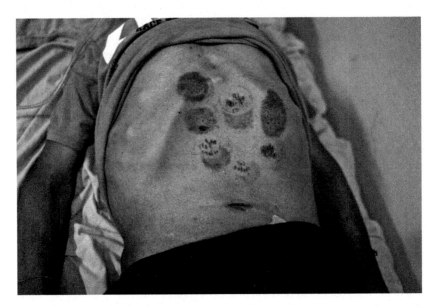

Illustration 1.6 Marks of Cutting and Sucking, *Mongar Hospital.* The markings on this man's stomach are similar to those incurred by Pema. The small red scars are a result of cutting with a razor blade, the larger red patches are caused by the vacuum when sucking through the ram's horn.

Finally, when the healer cuts Pema, the cure multiple, the practices that reinforce the becoming of health and body multiples, is enacted, completing a subjectivity of sorts, a patient amongst other patients. Conversely, her other bodies are enacted when the surgeon injects anaesthesia into her arm or the traditional-medicine pharmacist hands her the small bag of herbal pills. She becomes the body multiple in relation to the practices she enacts.

So on and so forth are bodies created, changed, lived, owned, claimed, destroyed, loved, abstracted and shared. Bhutan has many bodies, countless in their multiplicity, fleshy and social, feeling and unfelt, real, enacted and intense. Pema's breasts will give milk to her child, a sustenance body; in her office her fingers type on a keyboard, a technological body; her vagina walls exchange friction and electrical pulses to receive pleasure, a sexual body; her teeth grind food in a consumer body, a purchasing body, an energy body. A body is never singularly its flesh, bones, cartilage, not even its socio-cultural habitus, its economic utility, its political agenda. The bodies I encountered in Bhutan are multiples upon multiples, swarmed, coded and enacted in various forms that are beyond the comprehension and scope of those people that are these bodies, the powers that want to be these bodies and myself as an onlooker. This is our starting point, the 'unknowability' of bodies. There is no Totality of body-knowledge to be had, no Unity of a body, just collections of parts, body parts, sewn together numerous times by dynamic codification projects. These bodies rupture, parts detach, assembling new bodies continuously. To call this chaos is to value structure over default indeterminacy. It simply is, the body multiple.

The concept of the body multiple is not new. Annemarie Mol in her 2003 work *The Body Multiple: Ontology in Medical Practice* advances the work of many authors including Latour (1991), Strathern (1990 and 1992) and Hathaway (1990) to argue for a concept of multiple bodies, replacing a singular 'medical' object with a multiplicity of interrelated practices. Her ethnography describes how a vascular disease called atherosclerosis is 'done' in a Dutch hospital by patients, doctors and scientists. Within this tight biomedical setting, Mol uses vast empirical evidence to argue that the disease is multiplied by all the actors that enact it, ultimately producing multiple bodies in which these diseases reside.

Mol's work is philosophical in that it argues for an ontological position where objects, in this case the body and its disease, do not exist in and of themselves but rather in multiple 'enactments' of practices, diseases and knowledges. Commenting on her work, Jensen and Winthereik (2005: 266) note that 'this metaphysical standpoint is directly opposed to Kant's notion of das Ding an sich (the thing in itself) versus das Ding für uns (things as they are perceived). In the Kantian viewpoint, the relations that make up an object are somehow closed in on themselves and completely separable from the relations that "we" may forge with it. In Mol's view, the putative object "out there" is never closed in on itself. It is always constituted and re-constituted, i.e. enacted, in relation to various others.' The object of the body then emerges through multiple contingencies and is rendered multiple. I follow Mol's line of reasoning for the body and take the same approach to the 'patient', yet I discard claims to ontologies and rather focus the insights on the praxis of the body within social relations. Rather than philosophical claims, I assert that the body multiple is a performative strategy of patients like Pema to live fully in her world of diverse healthcare knowledges and practices.

This section has explained how Pema enacted her own body multiple through the bisecting of phenomenological experiences and the use of an alternative practice called 'cutting and sucking'. Following the two previous sections that explained both cure and health multiple, this third multiplicity concludes the constituent parts of what I argue as the 'patient multiple'.

Across Bhutan many other patients replicate Pema's process of body multiplication as they practice the diverse cure multiples available to them. Their bodies are bisected, interpreted and manipulated according to the various practices and healing knowledges they encounter. Each of these patients undergoes similar foregrounding by various health multiples that infuse knowledge contexts into the enactment processes. Right now, in hospital wards, healer's living rooms, pharmacies, traditional medicine units, bedrooms and monasteries across Bhutan, patients bodies, healths and cures are 'becoming' multiple.

Conclusion: Cohesive Multiples

This ethnography puts the patient in the foreground of all it explains. In each social network that it delves into, each assemblage, be it traditional medicine (chapter 2), decision-making (chapter 3), alternative practices (chapter 4) or medical materiality (chapter 5), the patient is placed at the front-end of examination. By doing so the patient becomes the nexus of conjoining themes. I take this methodological approach as it offers a starting point to a social subject that has no real origin. Health and the experience of it begins nowhere; it just planes outwards in continuously revolving cycles of becoming, over time, though space, materials and persons. But a text and a research must start somewhere. The patient offers a nodal location to begin fanning outwards to wider themes and details that will elucidate the ethnography. The patient focus also gives the ethnographer someone to talk to, someone with opinions, with actual becomings and experiences.

This chapter has built up to offering a working definition of what a 'patient' is within the healing contexts of Bhutan. It has done so by first presenting a snapshot of the health contexts of Bhutan that are navigated by persons seeking a cure. In exploring the different types of practices available to patients, we have come to understand the concept of 'cure multiple', a pluralistic ethnographic context of practice, entailing different technologies, knowledges and ethics. Next I discussed how patients, through the interaction with these cure multiples, enact multiple healths, where subjectivities are cascaded across multiple notions of what health is and how it is maintained or improved. Finally I argued that a patient has many bodies that are deployed in the contexts of both health and cure. These bodies have meaningful phenomenological experiences of pain and alleviation that go on to reinforce the multiples of health and practice.

I have used the example of a young woman who shared her healing narratives with me to demonstrate the processes of becoming a patient in Bhutan. Through close examination of the ethnographic evidence I arrived at the conclusion that on all three levels – cures, healths and bodies – Pema enacts a flexible multiplicity of patient subjectivities that inspire, effectuate and sustain healing. It is through this triadic understanding of cure, health and body multiple that I arrive at an applicable conception of 'patient multiple' that can be applied to the analysis of my ethnography at large. The patient multiple comprises these three dimensions. Pema is a patient multiple, a multi-subjectivity person who has different healths and bodies that are engaged in a diverse array of practices.

This conclusion raises ethnographic and theoretical difficulties: How does the patient retain coherency in the face of multiplicity? How can people stay sane in amongst such diversity of subjectivities? How does difference and contrast not cause destructive friction? Not once in my fieldwork did I meet a patient, a healthcare-seeking individual or community, who was overwhelmed by the diverse number of health service options available to them. Neither was there any sign of contestation between conceptions of health or even assemblages of medical knowledge. Patient multiplicity was accepted, encouraged and utilized effectively, and the question of coherency remained mute. How?

I would argue that multiple patient subjectivities and the practices that enact them offer an agentive meaningfulness to experiences of suffering and healing. Patients are often choosing for themselves which practices to use, which health a disease will inhabit, or which body to engage. Pema made this deliberate and aware decision when she visited the traditional hospital after the biomedical hospital. She also chose to visit an alternative healer for her stomach pain. These are lucid, informed and ultimately meaningful decisions that help her approach, understand and combat her illnesses. Even if the symptoms are not abated, the simple act of seeking healing through a particular patient subjectivity was rewarding and personally meaningful. When Pema felt her stomach ache and decided to seek the healer's remedy, she 'pivoted' into a particular patient subjectivity. It is this process of pivoting, the process of emergence, that brings agentive meaningfulness to healthcare-seeking; Pema was actioning against suffering, and this exertion of power and intent overrides differences between her patient multiples. Thus processes of enactment are themselves bonding, permitting cohesive persons amongst a multiplicity of subjectivities.

While the act of seeking healing may bring agentive meaningfulness to a patient, not all attempts at a cure succeed. Treatments can fail and patients can continue to suffer. What happens if a patient chooses a curative practice that doesn't work? What if they had chosen another that might have been more effective? Decision-making between practices can be meaningful to patients; it may keep them sane amongst diverse options, but it doesn't necessitate healing. Therefore, while choosing and enacting practices keeps the patient multiple cohesive, it may ultimately lead to the destruction of other bodies or subjectivities. In chapter 3 I explore these crucial moments of decision-making between curative trajectories and how these decisions might aid in maintaining and curing, as Pema tells us, 'one side' of a patient but not the other.

Notes

1. In instances of exact quotation recorded by digital recorder or handwritten notes, whether in English or translated from another language, I employ a simple grammar correction to allow an easier reading as well as to push focus on what was said and meant by the interviewee, rather than shrouding meaning in incorrect grammar. Where particular incorrect grammar constructs pointed to specific ethnographic detail, I have left this in the interview script so as not to lose this linguistic particularity.
2. See Kennedy 1985, Dale and Schaefer 2004, and Goroll and Mulley 2012: 1403–7 for more biomedical details on the diagnosis and treatment of sinusitis.
3. The phonetic follows the Dzongkha Development Commission's official romanisation of the term, rather than the THL Phonetic method, as used in global currency exchange markets.

4. This is the common way of spelling *ara* in its phonetic form in Bhutan as seen on many menus, signboards and bottles of alcohol. The THL Simple Phonetic transcription system would render this term *a rag*. However, I have opted for its more common and recognizable phonetic form.

5. In 1985, only 50 percent of Bhutan's population had primary healthcare coverage (MoH 1986: 5), a healthcare service that was much less developed than it is today. While these numbers may seem trivial, they are incredibly important for patient scenarios on the ground. For example, even with 90 percent coverage, this means 10 percent of the Bhutanese population doesn't have access to primary healthcare services. To empathize with this situation, imagine getting sick and not having any biomedical services to turn to – what would you do? This is still very much a problem faced by 10 percent of Bhutan's population.

6. The procurement of ambulances, two in each hospital, has been a major aim and financial undertaking for the Ministry of Health. The Japanese government donated approximately $1.5 million (*Nu* 98 million) in 2012 to achieve this goal (Ministry of Finance, MoF 2013: 19, 38)

7. For example, *Kuensel* Online (2013).

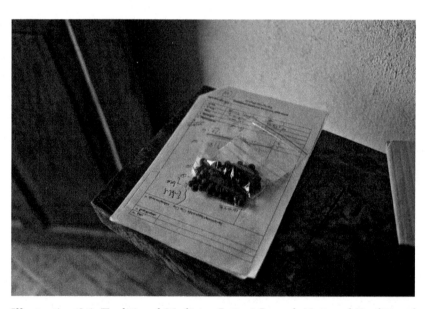

Illustration 2.1 Traditional-Medicine Patient Record, *National Traditional Medicine Hospital, Thimphu.* A patient's medicines rest on top of their yellow patient record sheet.

2

Modernizing Traditional Medicine
A Two-Option Healthcare Service

The Different Meanings of the Term 'Traditional Medicine'

The term 'traditional medicine' is used across the world to refer to a wide and changing array of medical practices often in juxtaposition to biomedicine. The World Health Organization (WHO) captures this generality well in its definition: 'Traditional medicine is the sum total of knowledge, skills and practices based on the theories, beliefs and experiences indigenous to different cultures that are used to maintain health, as well as to prevent, diagnose, improve or treat physical and mental illnesses' (WHO 2008). Medical industries, academics, international development agencies, governments and various other groups make use of this generality in applying the term to a vast array of practices, such as homeopathy, Ayurveda, Chinese medicine, marijuana use and acupuncture. The World Health Organization is one agency attempting to standardize this global diversity with its International Classification of Traditional Medicine scheme (WHO 2010 and Strafford 2011).

The term has also filtered into political and institutional agendas that seek traction through claims of authenticity and historicity, touting the benefits ascribed to 'traditional culture'. Such models of justification can be traced through philosophical and anthropological literature for some time. For example, Max Weber has described religious authorities, typically individuals, of power that are legitimized through a 'tradition' assumed sacred (1997: 359). DeLanda (2006: 68–93) is one of many to expand this idea into the legitimization of organizations through the replacement of individualized actors with organizational 'positions', powerful, but devoid of personalization, amassing to form an institutional network. These 'traditional' assemblages have 'many elements of rituals, like their choreography in space and time, that express legitimacy simply by conforming to past usage' (2006: 70). Craig (2012) and Prost (2008) bring ethnographic evidence to such processes within communities of Tibetan traditional medicine, showing how its proponents use the historicity of *sowa rigpa* to retain a sense of cultural and religious identity. Ultimately traditional medicine is more than just a practice; it enacts an epistemology, an identity and a position within a social or political context.

Accessible institutionalized medical services are a relatively new development in Bhutan. Before the 1960s there were only a handful of biomedical doctors, and the institutional forms of traditional medicine had yet to collectivize under the National Traditional Medicine Hospital (Malgaard and Dorji 2012: 53–70). While there were independent healers working in the rural communities, they worked privately as alternative practitioners do today. Without access to reliable medical clinics, the danger of sickness remained ever-present. Life expectancy has climbed from thirty-seven years in 1960 to sixty-seven in 2010 (World Bank 2013), a significant change that parallels the development of two-option state healthcare services beginning in the 1960s.

Today, Bhutanese patients have access to a two-option national healthcare service across the country, even in the most remote areas. Within many of these hospitals and clinics, patients have a choice between biomedical and traditional healthcare, both of which are institutions of the state.

This chapter explores what this 'traditional' type of medicine is, how it has institutionalized and how it goes on to affect patients that seek its diagnosis and treatment. By looking at the central hub of this traditional-medicine network, the National Traditional Medicine Hospital in Thimphu, and some of its external relations, I argue that through structured and deliberate processes of institutionalization, standardization and nationalization, traditional medicine is going on to create new forms of 'patient' and 'health' within individual and state levels.

Following the work of Petryna (2002) among others on 'biological citizenship', I conclude that these processes of patient creation within the institution of traditional medicine constitute what I call 'bio-traditional citizenship', a new emerging state category for a political and social subject, as defined by the Bhutanese knowledge and practice of *sowa rigpa*. Bhutan has had a long tradition of looking for innovative ways to develop and construct state identities that fall in line with a Buddhist philosophy (Ura and Penjore 2009; Allison 2004; Phuntsho 2004), and the policies of GNH is one case in point. I argue that traditional medicine services are creating a new type of national patient identity, one that promotes different notions of illness, health and body that call on a Buddhist or *sowa rigpa* knowledge. While in its infancy, such bio-traditional citizenship, with the aforementioned commitment to creative development strategies, could create a new way of envisioning national healthcare statistics and reporting, as well as the ways patients understand and navigate their own illnesses and healing in relation to state services. Such development trajectories will be critically important to sustaining traditional medicine within the two-option healthcare services, especially given biomedicine's dominancy thus far. It may also provide bridges to incommensurability between biomedicine and traditional medicine, helping the two practices better understand and incorporate one another.

In Bhutan the term 'traditional medicine' is often rearranged and used in different ways, similar to the international generality mentioned earlier. The category of traditional medicine is continually reassembled into multiples of practice, understanding and institutional forms. Patients, health workers, healers, administrators, businesses and other groups or persons may imply a complex of meanings in referencing a practice, medicine, aetiology, sickness or medical ideology. This linguistic diversity is housed in a plethora of terminology across the twenty-six languages of Bhutan, including English, which has its own linguistic currency. Examples of diversity in the use of the term 'traditional medicine' include its multiple translations, all employed to reference the institutionalized practice of the National Traditional Medicine Hospital: *nang pé men* (*nang pa'i sman*, traditional medicine[1]), *nang pé ga man* (Shr: traditional medicine), *sowa rigpa* (the art and science of Buddhist healing), Indigenous Medicine (Eng: the former term for traditional medicine, occasionally still used as a formal term), and *drukpa men* ('*brug pa sman*, Bhutanese medicine). The term 'traditional medicine' is also transmuted and applied in different grammatical ways; for example, a patient might refer to a 'traditional disease', or a health administrator might call a particular treatment a 'traditional practice'.

While these terms may be used to reference specifically the National Traditional Medicine Hospital, they are also used to refer to what I call 'alternative practices'. These are non-institutionalized practices that are not a part of the National Traditional Medicine Hospital yet were sometimes collapsed linguistically into or onto one another, taking the form 'traditional practices'. On the third floor of the Ministry of Health, in the office of the Health and Religion programme responsible for, in the ministry's terms, some of the more 'cultural and religious' aspects of medicine, I sat with two senior officers, discussing the variants of these non-institutionalized alternative practices found in Bhutan. They are responsible for writing the policy and training documents concerning what they called 'traditional healers' distributed to national health staff, including *drungtsho* and *menpa*. I was presented with the 'Traditional Healers Training Guideline' (MoH 2011c), a manual on how to encourage the adaption of 'modern' safety protocols into these healers' activities. The two officers agreed that these 'traditional healers' should be rigorously monitored and registered. I asked them who should be registered. They told me those who do 'traditional medicine', like the healers who do 'cutting and sucking' or bone setting. They pointed to a list included in the text. 'What about the *drungtsho* in the Thimphu National Traditional Medicine Hospital?' I asked. They paused for a moment to think as the categorizations became more complex, and then one told me that 'traditional medicine is okay, it's registered. It's the other traditional medicine that's dangerous.'

In this context, 'traditional medicine' was defined by a government institution capable of applying different definitions of the term to governing policies and protocols. This office is central to how the Ministry of Health labels and then interacts with the large number of alternative healers, including shamans, *lamas*, bone setters, *pawo* and *pamo*, and *ja né* healers (see chapter 4). Given the complex and constantly evolving practices that these healers perform, the ministry has yet to rigidly classify each practice, leaving the cluster of practices and practitioners to break apart and reformulate depending on the institutional agendas.

Months later, I sat next to a forty-year-old taxi driver as he whirled me around the winding streets of Motithang, a northern district of Thimphu where I lived. I often took these opportunities to conduct small interviews or discussions regarding my latest ethnographic enquiry. This particular conversation was in Dzongkha, but it could have been in any three of the languages – Dzongkha, English and Nepali – I could converse in. He asked me, as everyone always did, what I was doing in Bhutan.

> JONATHAN: I'm a *nang pé men* [traditional medicine] researcher.
> TAXI DRIVER: A what?
> JONATHAN: I am a student studying *sowa rigpa*.
> TAXI DRIVER: What's that?
> JONATHAN: It's a type of medicine. I work with *drungtsho* in the *nang pé men khang* [traditional medicine hospital].
> TAXI DRIVER: Where?
> JONATHAN: The traditional-medicine hospital. [In English, used purposely to see if he understands].
> TAXI DRIVER: [A quizzical facial expression]
> JONATHAN: You know, the hospital just down the hill, close to the UNICEF office.
> TAXI DRIVER: Oh yes, the Drukpa *men khang* [Bhutanese medicine hospital]. I take Drukpa *men* every day.

He reached into the front pocket of his *gho* and pulled out a small plastic ziplock bag with a few Dzongkha scribbles on it and some brown tablets inside, typical of those given from the dispensary at the Drukpa *men khang*, or in other terms the National Traditional Medicine Hospital. 'Drukpa *men* cures the cause of my illness, and it's natural', he said, as did so many of my interviewees when asked about the positives of traditional medicine. The taxi pulled up outside the Drukpa *men khang* and I got out.

While biomedicine is often seen as coming from 'outside' of the country, practices falling under the nomenclature of traditional medicine often have a locational specificity within or of Bhutan. This may relate to the nation-state as seen earlier, or with more 'local' orientations, including geographies, communities and cultural or ethnic identities. From such spatial orientation comes the prefix 'local' to the terms 'healer', 'medicine' or 'practice', commonly used interchangeably with the prefix 'traditional'. Thus 'Drukpa *men*', literally translated as 'Bhutanese medicine', can be applied to a vast number of practices ascribed to a locality within Bhutan and its cultural landscape.

Linguistic ambiguity continues even in the national press. On 17 April 2012, the Bhutan Broadcast Service (BBS), the biggest media outlet in Bhutan, released a story entitled 'Traditional Medicines Seized from a Local Practitioner.' The story read, 'After a search warrant, the inspectors of Drug Regulatory Authority today searched and seized some 90 packets of traditional medicine from a local medical practitioner in Semtokha, Thimphu. It was reported that a Bhutanese living in Geneva [Switzerland] suffered from lead poisoning after taking medicine from the practitioner. At the end of last year, he visited Thimphu and took the traditional medicine from the local medical practitioner, a monk, to treat facial nerve palsy. And in two months' time, he was admitted in one of the hospitals in Geneva with acute pain in the stomach and right side of the abdomen' (BBS 2012d). The 'local practitioner' was fined *Nu*18,900 (approximately USD$340) and signed a letter of undertaking stating that he would stop his practice. The Drug Regulatory Authority, the Ministry of Health and Menjong Sorig Pharmacuticals, the producers of traditional medicine used in the national traditional health services, along with most media outlets, deemed this 'traditional medicine' a poison.

The singular term of 'traditional medicine' may then reference a multitude of different practices, even by state-run media. The term is so prolifically used in different linguistic variations by a wide range of people or social groups all over the country that attempts at categorizing or defining the different instances of use could undermine the agency of the term itself, for its mutability in application gave the speaker a flexibility of expression while remaining referentially ambiguous. This ambiguity is important to many patients, as it offers a dynamic mode of expression that can help in discussing pain, sickness causality and healing practices. If 'traditional medicine' may refer to any number of practices, ideologies or epistemologies, then the patient is presented with a more vast and non-contradictory potential for expression. Such transmutability helps maintain 'coherency' in the face of patient multiplicity, as argued for in the conclusion of chapter 1.

While definitional variance in the term 'traditional medicine' is the norm, it is clear that it never references the biomedical services offered by the government. Biomedicine is by far the most prolifically used medicine in Bhutan, with the ministry reporting a total of 1,990,958 cases availing its nationwide services in 2012 (MoH 2013a: 66), more than double the 750,000 population of Bhutan. In the face of such a widely used practice, any healing technique different from biomedical services falls into a position of disassociation. This is an important terminological distinction, whereby disassociation from biomedicine creates space for a different cluster of practices; in the case of Bhutan, the term 'traditional medicine' has become a placeholder for this opposing position, whether or not it refers to institutionalized or non-institutionalized practices.

Processes of Becoming a Traditional-Medicine Institution

Institutional Body Functions

With the acknowledgement of linguistic mutability, there does arise one assemblage of healing practice that is increasing its foothold across the medical landscape in Bhutan due to its adoption and propagation by the Royal Government of Bhutan, the Ministry of Health, the Dzongkha Development Commission (DDC) and the National Traditional Medicine Hospital. This practice has its foundations in *sowa rigpa* and is known by the ministry and those who practice it as *nang pé men* or 'traditional medicine', and I will use these terms interchangeably henceforth to refer only to this particular practice. However, the term 'traditional' does not allude to a temporal antiquity of the institution or its practice. What is described is a 'modern' institution of traditional medicine in a perpetual mode of evolution and change, and arguably one that is 'newer' than its biomedical counterpart.

In 1958, with medical practitioners and administrators just beginning to institutionalize, the third king, Jigme Dorji Wangchuk, and the newly formed National Assembly initiated the organization of a traditional-medicine school in Bhutan (National Assembly of Bhutan 1958: 3). This school built upon the knowledge and practices of a few *nang pé men drungtsho* that treated royalty and any patients lucky enough to gain access to them.[2] Following what had been a slow and sporadic introduction of a practice inherited from Tibet, this resolution and school marked the beginning of a professionalization, nationalization and standardization process that continues in the institutionalized forms of traditional medicine in Bhutan.

This original school is now the Faculty of Traditional Medicine (FTM), formally the National Institute of Traditional Medicine (NITM, founded in 1971 as the Training Centre for Indigenous Medicine), and it trains *drungtsho* (physicians) and *menpa* (clinical assistants), awarding bachelor's degrees and diplomas in traditional medicine for respective professions. Matriculating students are registered with the Bhutan Medical and Health Council, which is responsible for certifying all medical practitioners in the country, and go on to take positions in nationwide clinics. The institution has many similarities to a biomedical-medicine school, with a core curriculum, entrance and final qualification examinations, a full-time faculty, residency placements and Bhutan Medical and Health Council–approved certification courses ranging from five years for *drungtsho* to three years for *menpa*. While the structure is similar to biomedical-school models, the institute's curriculum, teaching methods and examinations are markedly different, focusing more on some of the formal *sowa rigpa* training methods; for example, *drungtsho* have to memorize and recite the four major Buddhist medical texts, the *gyü zhi*.[3] The Faculty of Traditional Medicine is officially affiliated with the Royal University of Bhutan (RUB) due to efforts by the government to house all public training institutes under one administrative board.

Graduating *nang pé men* professionals are positioned within the National Traditional Medicine Hospital (NTMH 2007). This institution is responsible for the administration and delivery of patient services, both in Thimphu and throughout the growing number of service locations nationwide, known to the ministry and the National Traditional Medicine Hospital as 'traditional-medicine units'. The National Traditional Medicine Hospital is a clinical and training institution and hosts the administrative unit staffed mostly by *sowa rigpa*–trained *drungtsho* and *menpa*. In 2012 the hospital treated 49,527 cases, with the nationwide clinics treating a total of 131,692 cases (the NTMH included; MoH 2013a: 98). The institution falls under the purview of the Ministry of Health and is included in its administration, budgeting, monitoring and reporting as one of the growing 'units' in the ministry's health services. Currently the hospital is entering a new phase of representation and political agency in the ministry with its recent (November 2011) elevation to 'Division' status and an anticipated forthcoming further development into a 'Department'. Such changes will elevate the administrative powers of the National Traditional Medicine Hospital, an organizational development that is deemed necessary by the heads of the administrative sections of the hospital to meet the growing patient demands in Thimphu and throughout the rest of the country.

The third branch of the *nang pé men* services is named Menjong Sorig Pharmaceuticals (MSP) as of December 2011, formally known as the Pharmaceutical Research Unit (PRU). Menjong Sorig Pharmaceuticals produces eight to ten metric tons of the ninety-eight traditional medicines that are distributed to clinics nationwide. They are responsible for the collecting, processing and testing of raw materials, as well as interfacing with the Drug Regulatory Authority to timely meet supply demands. They also produce a range of commercial and religious products using raw materials found on Bhutan's mountainsides, such as Tseringma herbal tea and *ril bu* (*ril bu*), the small black pills used in religious ceremonies. From the early 1950s medicines were usually made by the *drungtsho* themselves, either in collaboration with their colleagues in their respective clinics or independently. Mechanization was scarce until 1982 when the World Health Organization contributed some basic grinding equipment to the small cottage factory. In 1994 the European Union committed to a multiphase project to fully mechanize the manufacturing process, along with the construction of a larger factory building that now stands at the entrance to the traditional medicine compound in Thimphu. Today the medicines are produced mostly by trained workers and a series of machines. Quality assurance testing is performed onsite as are research and development, marketing and administration.

In 1998 these three institutions were unified under a single name, the Institute of Traditional Medicine Services, and were affiliated with the Ministry of

Health. However, as of 2011, this structure was retired for a more independent model that saw each institution move under a different umbrella of the Royal Government of Bhutan. While they remain separate from an organizational point of view, they are co-dependent on each other and thus remain in close cooperation.

Enacting the Institution through Centralized Pressures and Demands

At the centre of the expansion of traditional medicine in Bhutan is the National Traditional Medicine Hospital, a national health institution with two major functions. The first is to clinically diagnose and treat patients under its adopted practice of *nang pé men*, using a set of standardized therapy practices that give the hospital its reputation amongst its patients.[4] The second is to administer the nationwide traditional medicine units, a task that is growing ever more difficult given the rapid expansion of units, patients and graduating *drungtsho* and *menpa*. Both of these functions are performed by *nang pé men* – trained civil servants, most of whom graduated from the Faculty of Traditional Medicine and are registered *drungtsho* or *menpa*; the only practitioners to not have graduated from the institute would be some of the senior staff whose training preceded the foundation of the college.

As of September 2013 the hospital employed fifty-one people: twelve *drungtsho*, twenty-two *menpa*, fourteen administration staff, two cleaners and one museum caretaker.

At the back of the hospital compound stands the administrative block, a long thin wooden structure with an open-air walkway offering access to the low-ceiling offices that are crammed with computers, printers and filing cabinets. Until the mid-1990s this building was the medicine-production unit; then the EU's funding arrived to build the factory across from the compound. Although this block is rustic and may appear unappealing to first-time visitors, these offices house some of the most important characters in the traditional medicine hospital: administrative officers who perform a wide range of tasks that steer the activities, production and expansion of traditional medical services across the country. I would often visit them, interrupting the writing of a ministry proposal, a monitoring report, a standard practice manual, a medicine restocking order or other important document written in English or Dzongkha. The officers in this building are mostly trained *menpa*, but due to their computer literacy and English comprehension they are enlisted to construct bureaucratic and institutional texts, a key component to the transparency, validation and growth of a government institution in Bhutan. They have also developed a certain level of political savviness and institutional poise, a requirement for an effectual day's administrative work. The offices may be empty as these *menpa* often attend meetings or deliver documents to the ministry.

The administrators of the hospital and nationwide units are trained *nang pé men* clinicians, not hospital or health system administrators.[5] This poses a challenge as the traditional-medicine services enter a new decade of growth and accompanying scrutiny, increasing the need for health system management, as demanded by the Ministry of Health, biomedical doctors and international organizations like the World Health Organization or United Nations Development Program. These stakeholders want traditional medicine to meet national health issues in an effective and transparent manner. A Bhutanese surgeon made the point clear over dinner one evening: 'Okay, traditional medicine can help treat a few chronic illnesses effectively, but can it meet the demands of our national health problems, like diabetes, HIV and liver disease? If not, should it be so heavily funded by the government?' Most biomedical professionals like this surgeon have much respect for traditional medicine – they often say that their own mothers use the practice with their encouragement – but they voice openly their concerns of its effectiveness in the face of national health issues. The traditional hospital has produced one study of efficacy (Singye 2012), yet this does not amount to the demands for an evidence-based report as desired by the doctor. While there is much debate regarding the applicability of evidence-based research to *nang pé men*, there is mounting pressure for the services to demonstrate the curative properties of traditional medicine and to meet public demand. It is up to the *nang pé men*–trained administrators to meet these demands and show that the practice is addressing national health concerns.

I asked many people involved in overseeing the hospital about the option to hire administrators trained in healthcare management and not *nang pé men*. Caution was voiced towards other education models, with many preferring a foundation first in *nang pé men* and then additional training in hospital management. Requiring *nang pé men* for hospital administrative staff marks one part of a multifaceted effort to maintain as much influence and direction from traditional medicine as possible. The fear of many who work in the traditional-medicine administrative and clinical units is that modern biomedical influences will invade *nang pé men* and dilute its already struggling philosophies, practices and theory at both management and practice levels. Another example of this would be the decisive use of Dzongkha in institutional writing and communication, rather than English as used by most civil service institutions, to maintain an 'essence' of *nang pé men* that is lost in English translation. The ministry kindly receives these communiqués in Dzongkha, but English versions are often attached or later requested if the memo and its agenda are to be continued. The invasions of modernity into the traditional is a dialectic tug-of-war that continually resurfaces as social, political and economic resources are assembled for various purposes, including traditional medicine, alternative healing practices or biomedicine. However, efforts to diversify and modernize on-the-job training are ongoing. For example, I was asked to identify a six-month international training course in hospital management, preferably based in London, to which two *drungtsho* might be sent. While the courses were deemed too expensive, the effort demonstrates an increased interest to incorporate biomedical health-care management techniques into *nang pé men* services.

The largest building of the hospital, which walls three sides of the central courtyard, houses the consultation rooms, dispensary, a few therapy rooms and the reception window. The offices of the medical superintendent and chief administrator are also situated up a narrow wooden staircase on the second floor. This structure is constructed primarily from wood and painted in the Bhutanese tradition, giving an older and softer sensory experience than many of the concrete hospitals and BHUs around the country. Patients gather in the open-air corridors between the hospital rooms and the courtyard awaiting their turn for a *drungtsho* consultation or one of the many therapies on offer.

Across the courtyard a crowd often gathers by two large spinning prayer wheels. They sit and chat, awaiting their medications. Inside the dispensary, up to four sets of quick hands take yellow prescription sheets from the window and fill small plastic ziplock bags with an assortment of pills. There is a constant frenetic rush to meet the demands for medicines. On a busy day, the *menpa* may fill over three hundred prescriptions, a tiresome task that has them standing on their feet all day. Comparatively in the consultation rooms, where I spent most of my time observing patient-*drungtsho* interactions, the pace of work is calmer, except on the mornings of Saturday and Monday when patients simultaneously converge on the hospital, causing long queues outside the chambers. Some *drungtsho* operate a first-come, first-served queuing system; others leave it to the sharp and persistent elbows of waiting patients.

Processes of Becoming a Traditional Medicine Patient

Across a National Network

An elderly female patient sat quietly on a stiff wooden bench in the corridors of the National Traditional Medicine Hospital in Thimphu. The waiting area is part of a three-sided inner courtyard that forms the central hub of the hospital. It has no walls and is thus exposed to the weather of the day. The open space allows all to see who is waiting for what room, what specialty of treatment, or which *drungtsho*, a senior, a chief, a new trainee, an assistant or a *menpa*. While waiting is a spectacle, the *drungtsho* chambers are kept private by heavy swinging doors, protected by its occupants who allow only one patient in at a time. It was hot. The sun beat down on our backs that were turned to the courtyard. The elderly patient's full *kira* looked stifling, so much so that as I sat next to her I could see the sweat beading around the metal chain necklace that hung around her neck. She waited to see the most senior *drungtsho* in the hospital, chamber number one.

In her hands she held two materials. Her right hand clasped a *mala* (*cheng ma, 'phreng ma*) necklace, flipping the beads rhythmically one by one. I sensed a nervousness, a hoping, a desire for amelioration. Religiosity intertwined with medical intervention. She held a pile of yellow papers in her left hand that looked as though they had been scrunched up, rubbed in mud then ironed flat in an attempt at formal presentation. Each page of this bundle of medical records held information on either a traditional or biomedical service. These forms were designed and printed in Thimphu by the Ministry of Health and distributed nationwide; the blank forms could be found on any doctor's desk or reception area in Bhutan's healthcare centres. I asked to see them. She was willing and thrust them at me; in the early 1900s when the first British officers of the Indian Medical Service began journeying into Bhutan by foot, they were often met by throngs of patients demanding a foreigner's panacea (see McKay 2007 or White 1984). A sentiment of this continues in present day; even if a traditional-medicine prescription is written in shorthand Dzongkha it would often end up in my hands for review.

The shorthand text on these pages dated back a few years and told a story of this patient's quest for a cure. She would hand the narrative to the *drungtsho* in chamber one so that he could assess years of sickness and pain in a quick five-minute consultation. The first page showed a diagnosis and prescription that was given to her by a *drungtsho* visiting her small village in the eastern Trashiyangtse *dzongkhag*, two days walk from the nearest road head, a four-day journey to Thimphu. *Drungtsho* across Bhutan occasionally go on tour to remote locations, often with a biomedical team, packing a few basic medications and offering consultations for those unable or unwilling to make the walk to the nearest health clinic. In this first instance, a practitioner and a medicine had come to her. With this doctor came a diagnosis for her disease, one specific to the logic and knowledge of *sowa rigpa*,and encoded with a *nang pé men* 'disease code', a concept explored further in the next section. This coded diagnosis was meaningless to the patient who couldn't read its encryption. But for the next *drungtsho* she would see, it would lay the foundation for the treatments to follow.

The second page was an English biomedicine form listing paracetamol, prescribed by a 'health assistant' who worked at the BHU staged at the road head. No traditional doctor was available there so she had settled with his prescription. There are only 35 *drungtsho* and 63 *menpa* (MoH 2013a: 109) in Bhutan, with 254 BHUs to staff. Biomedical services filled most of the service posts in these more remote locations. With the walking portion of the journey made, it was now only a seven-hour car or bus ride to the next health post she wanted to visit in Mongar.

The third page was headed 'Mongar Eastern Regional Referral Hospital, Traditional Medicine Unit', the second biggest hospital in the country, serving patients in the eastern *dzongkhags*. There are two *drungtsho* and two *menpa* there, along with a wider variety of medicines and treatment options. She stayed a week somewhere close to the hospital; the form didn't say where or with whom – it never did. This information is beyond the scope of the form's twelve information fields. Gaps in the patient narrative are everywhere, but they are necessary – they create space for what can be known about the patient. More traditional medicine was given to her by the Mongar *drungtsho*, as were steam-bath treatments, where she lay on a wooden bed boxed in by a suspended blue sheet as herbal steam was pumped into the chamber. These treatments were described on the third page, which then ended with a referral note to the Thimphu traditional hospital. The hierarchy of treatment options spread out across pages, an order of perceived effectiveness that patients are so often aware of and seek to pursue. This patient decided to make the two-day journey across the country by bus.

She now sat, waiting to see a more senior *drungtsho*, one who had practiced for longer and might be able to read her pulse more accurately; *drungtsho* and patients both agree that the longer one practices, the more subtle and acute one's tactile abilities become for pulse reading. This senior *drungtsho* might also offer her a more specialized medication unavailable in any of the other clinics. There are medications on the shelves of the Thimphu dispensary – accessed only through the *drungtsho*'s scribbled prescription – that cannot be found elsewhere in the country. There is a hierarchy of available medications in relation to the type of clinic, dictated by a continually evolving document called the 'Essential Drugs List' (DRA 2013b), published by the Ministry of Health for both traditional and biomedical medicines. She waited in the sun, fully aware of these healing potentials. Her right and left hands moved anxiously together, thumbing beads and paper, becoming religiosity and medical narratives, fostering hope.

This story demonstrates the access patients have to traditional medicine across Bhutan in a variety of different capacities and locations. Patients who visit health centres are faced with a 'traditional'-medicine option, which is now a viable and accessible response to suffering, even for those living in remote areas. As of 2011 there were forty-six traditional units, including one national referral hospital, one regional unit in Mongar Hospital and forty-four district hospital or BHU clinics, with an average of one *drungtsho* and one *menpa* per unit. Figure 2.1 shows the growth of these units since 1985, when only five units operated, as well as the growing number of *drungtsho* and *menpa*.

As the number of units has increased along with the knowledge of traditional-medicine practice among the general populace, the number of patients has increased. To meet these demands, the training of traditional-medicine staff by the Faculty of Traditional Medicine has accelerated, especially for *menpa*. Note in figure 2.1 that *menpa* exceeded the number of *drungtsho* for the first time in 2003, a balance shift that represents the growth of the institute and the need for more at-hand staff to fulfil administrative and clinical duties for the increasing number of nationwide units and patients.

Monitoring and reporting the figures of patients visiting traditional-medicine units is tracked by the National Traditional Medicine Hospital and its nationwide branches. Monthly reports are sent to the Thimphu hospital to be collated and annually presented in the Ministry of Health's publication, the

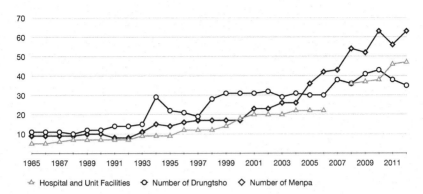

Figure 2.1 Number of Traditional-Medicine Staff and Facilities from 1985 to 2012. Source: Data collated from Ministry of Health Annual Health Bulletins from 1985 to 2012.

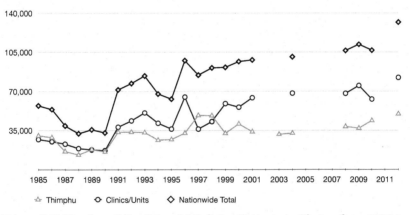

Figure 2.2 Number of Traditional-Medicine Patients in Bhutan from 1985 to 2012. Source: Data collated from Ministry of Health Annual Health Bulletins from 1985 to 2012.

Annual Health Bulletin (MoH 1986 to 2015). Figure 2.2 shows the growth in the number of traditional-medicine patients since 1985, when tracking patient figures began. As already stated, in 2012 the National Traditional Medicine Hospital reported 131,692 patient visits across its forty-nine units, with 49,527 of these being seen in the Thimphu hospital (MoH 2013a: 99).

Considering Bhutan's population of approximately 750,000, this means that about 14 percent, or at least one in ten people, used traditional-medicine services in 2010. Given the available data, this is a percentage that has continuously increased since 1985 and is most likely a trend that will continue given the further expansion of traditional-medicine services to more remote locations and its growing exposure in public health initiatives.

One way of viewing the dispersal and growth of a medical knowledge and practice amongst a population was described by Petryna (2002) in her account of patients' struggles to gain effective treatment in the wake of the 1986 Chernobyl disaster. She explains the idea of 'biological citizenship', a body-state category that uses biomedical markers to identify eligible patients for treatment and, in doing so, assembles nation-state citizens within this biomedical network. In Petryna's ethnography we see patients encoding themselves within these biological citizenship identities to gain access to state services. Cooper (2012), in her recent dissertation on medicine and citizenship in Venezuela, makes a similar argument from her ethnographic data, claiming that Venezuelan citizenship has become 'medically mediated' (2013: 6), transforming healing into a 'political experience of citizenship' (2013: 73). Many other medical anthropologists have followed suit with this argument, claiming biological and medical identities as integral to contemporary citizenship (along with Petryna 2008, see e.g. Rose and Miller 1992; Rose and Novas 2008; or Rabinow and Rose 2006). Patients in Bhutan are exposed to similar types of biological citizenship, whereby access to treatments is dependent on the fusion between medical and state identities.

A particularly poignant example of this can be seen in the Ministry of Health's international referral programme. Bhutanese patients that suffer from ailments that Bhutan's biomedical services are unable to treat – for example, leukemia or chronic hepatitis – are offered a fully paid trip to India to receive treatment. To be eligible for such an expensive referral, patients must present their biomedical and citizenship records to a Ministry of Health committee, who assesses their health and citizenship status. The latter often proves contentious, especially if a patient's parents were not born in Bhutan or the patient does not have full citizenship for other reasons. Given the massive expense of this programme (approximately *Nu*134 million, £1.6 million, in 2010, equating to 6 percent of the annual health budget; MoH 2011e: 24) and the limited allocation of resources to the large demand, it is difficult for patients who don't meet the selection criteria to access treatment abroad. Such a referral programme, and the political-medical identities it engenders, is a method of creating biological citizenship, specifically within the biomedical sphere of healthcare in Bhutan. Traditional-medicine services are excluded from this referral programme but not from other processes of biological citizenship.

The increase in *nang pé men* patients and the growth of the institution, as evidenced by the data presented and the story of the elderly woman seeking referral across a national network of clinics, demands that the idea of the biological citizen, as discussed by Petryna and others, be expanded to include a *nang pé men* dimension. 'Biological' is no longer synonymous with 'biomedical'. Patient demand is up from ten years ago, across both biomedical and traditional services. As one doctor told me, 'We used to have to beg for patients to come and use our services; now too many are coming and they are demanding services from us!' A new medical-state consciousness is developing among patients, where patrons of the state have a right to medical services for free. These patients are seeking, demanding and requesting services from their state, and in doing so they are assembling new forms of bio-traditional citizens (or bio–*nang pé* citizens). This process of becoming occurs with every *nang pé men* consultation and accompanying patient record sheet, explored in the next section.

Consultation

A patient may arrive at a hospital by taxi, private car or motorcycle, or on foot. Without a city bus service, patients rely on taxis as the predominant mode of travel for those without a vehicle. Private vehicle ownership is increasing daily in Thimphu with cars becoming a coveted and sought-after item (Ministry of Information and Communication 2011). However, the travel arrangements of patients, the distance travelled and the mode of transportation has little to do with the hospital. Unlike the biomedical-medicine services, traditional-medicine clinics offer outpatient services only, and they have no ambulance; therefore, patients are responsible for getting to and from the hospital. In many cases the *drungtsho* office is the spatial marker of 'inside' or 'outside' of the hospital purview. With many patients lining up outside her office, one female *drungtsho* doesn't have the time to track cases further than the seat opposite her desk. The patient record sheet she uses to list patient complaints and prescriptions in detail is supposed to do this job. Thus the patient seat becomes an important space-time marker in the patient's relationship and experience with the institution, whereby it is the only opportunity for personal consultation and diagnostic decision-making. Before and beyond this position, the patient is connected with the institution through various relations of exteriority, including but not limited to materials such as record sheets or medicines.

I am told by many of the elder *drungtsho* that this wasn't always the case. Before the number of patients increased and patient consultations became more formalized, patient-*drungtsho* relationships would extend beyond the hospital lines, with *drungtsho* visiting sick patients and their families in their homes. I was told there was a greater capacity for care beyond the consultation room, and *drungtsho* would and could use more personal social networks to care for their patients, whether they arranged accommodation, a carer, transportation or meal provision. However, these more 'personalized' practices are becoming scarce as patient demands and protocols to meet these demands increase in the institution of *nang pé men*. This is a transition in process evidenced between the different generations of *drungtsho*. Younger *drungtsho* in the hospital don't have much time for patients outside of the consultation room. They practice 'by the book'. The elder *drungtsho* take a more social approach. For example, patients might spend longer in these offices as they discuss non-medical gossip. Oftentimes in chamber one or two (the senior *drungtsho* offices), patients,

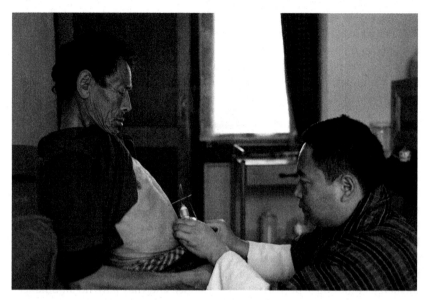

Illustration 2.2 Golden Needle Treatment, *National Traditional Medicine Hospital, Thimphu.* The golden needle is heated and then pressed against the skin, which pops and cracks as it blisters. The *drungtsho* will target the needle on either pain locations or on specific body points relating to energy lines as understood in *sowa rigpa*, similar to those of Chinese acupuncture. After a day of golden needle therapy, popular amongst patients, the room is filled with smoke and smells like burnt skin.

friends and families are seated for a group consultation or chat. But the elder *drungtsho* are retiring. One of the more senior *drungtsho* who hung up his white coat during my first few months in Thimphu told me that he continues to see loyal patients at home who have been under his care for decades. These senior *drungtsho* have seen the transition from 'informal' to 'formal' and carry with them ways of practice that are fading.

On arrival at the hospital, patients first visit the small reception window at the entrance of the hospital. The window is small and low, causing most people to hunch forwards and crane their necks backwards to greet the inhabitants inside the dark and bare office. The receptionist asks for previous record sheets. After an initial historical assessment, they direct the patient to a particular chamber number for consultation or therapy. If it's a returning patient, they will visit the *drungtsho* they met previously so that he or she may follow up with the case and offer a referral if necessary. New patients are given a clean patient record sheet and sent to either chamber seven or eight, where a junior *drung-tsho* is available for an initial consultation.

The inside of the nine consultation rooms is mostly alike except for a few differences that take particular medical specialties into account (Nidup 2009), such as steam treatment (*lang dug, slang dug,* Choden 2009), golden needle therapy (*tra den ser khap, spra gden gser khab,* T. Wangchuk 2009) or blood-letting (*tar, gtar,* Wangdi 2008). A large desk usually covered with papers, books or a computer juts into the centre of the small room, with a sink, a patient examination bed, a cabinet and a few extra seats taking up the rest of the space. The natural light fades as it hits the small and cloudy glass windows, causing a dim, grey-lit interior. Fading white paint is occasionally covered by a hospital memo stamped and signed with all the correct symbols. In one room a large public health poster of a mother and child with the words 'Take Antibiotics Responsibly' hangs above the desk where patients have their pulses read for humoural imbalances, possibly from negative karmic action or from environmental factors such as erroneous drug consumption.

While each chamber acts as a consultation room, some have additional equipment for specific medical treatments. The two steam-treatment rooms have wooden beds with a lower chamber below them for water boilers. A blue sheet covers the beds and the patients to box in the rising steam. Next to these are two wetrooms with makeshift bathtubs for herbal baths. The golden needle therapy room was immediately identifiable by a burning kerosene lamp, a needle held by medical pliers and the stench of burning skin. The bloodletting room was less obvious; all the practice requires is a tourniquet, usually made with cotton material and a bamboo stick, and a small blade, all kept in a desk drawer or cupboard.

What happened when I met Pema (see chapter 1) for the first time is a good example of how patients enter chambers. The opening of the spring-loaded door signalled her to rise from the hard wooden bench and squeeze past the departing patient. I craned my neck to see Pema enter respectfully, back hunched, head slightly bowed, hands and arms tight to the body, eyes downward, movements slow and cautious. The seat next to the desk remained empty until the *drungtsho* invited her to sit. She sat quietly until the *drungtsho* smiled and asked her why she had come.

This timidity in approach is a ritual of respect given to doctors, *drungtsho* and healers, and it was something I saw many patients in both traditional and biomedical clinics enact regularly. Practitioners are gateways to healthiness who hold much specialized knowledge, thus there was a need for an exchange: respect was offered in turn for amelioration. However, this coy approach was not always the norm: a friend of the *drungtsho,* a dignitary or more confident patient might approach the *drungtsho* in a more brazen and assertive fashion. Outside of this performative space, patients may also talk more freely about *drungtsho* or health professionals, asserting opinions on effectiveness or quality. Thus *drungtsho* and doctor authority and respect enacted itself on a sliding scale of intensity dependent on the configuration of relationships and social spacing.

The theory of *nang pé men* as applied in the classrooms of the Faculty of Traditional Medicine instills in its students methods of observation, examination and questioning (Leytho 2009). Similar to biomedicine, one follows a systematic checklist, ideally surveying the totality of a patient's health. The diagnostic root of the *sowa rigpa* practice memorized by students includes three 'trunks': visual observation, including tongue and urine inspection, pulse reading and questioning. Each of these diagnostic tools aims to uncover the balance between the wind (*lung, rlung*), bile (*tripa, mkhis pa*) and phlegm (*bé ken, bad kan*) humours. A disruption or agitation in one or more of the humours results in disease and sickness (Nidup 2010). The observation process begins when the patient is first met. The *drungtsho* will survey the complexion of the skin, the general mood of the patient and any other visual clues that may relate to the health state. When the patient is seated, the *drungtsho* will begin the questioning.

The questions aim to uncover the symptoms suffered and the behaviours or contexts surrounding the patient's complaints. *Nang pé men* breaks the questioning into three lines of inquiry, one for each humour. Each humour is associated with specific dietary, behavioural and pain qualities, and humoural imbalances can be identified by exploring the ways in which these associations are embedded in a patient's life. For example, Bhutan has a high incidence of chronic liver damage and stomach ulcers due to the dangerous dietary cocktail of strong alcohol and the most popular vegetable, the chilli (in 2012, Bhutan had an increasing incidence rate of twenty-nine per ten thousand for people suffering from alcohol-related liver disease; MoH 2012: 18). These two ailments, recognized by *nang pé men*, are bile-related diseases. If a patient complains about stomach pains, the *drungtsho* might ask, 'Do you drink strong alcohol? Does your mouth taste bitter? Do you eat many chillies? Does your body feel hot?' Positive answers would signify an aggravated bile humour and point to liver damage or a stomach ulcer, if not both.

After a series of questions the *drungtsho* then takes the patient's pulse. As the patient's forearm rests on the desk, the *drungtsho* uses the tactile function of their three forefingers to analyze the pulses of blood coursing through veins (see figure 2.3. They feel for discrepancies between beats, fading strengths, undulations of upthrusts, and constancy within each pulse's oscillation. While much has already been written on the art of pulse reading in the *sowa rigpa* practice,[6] a short description of it here will help intimate some of the theories of *sowa rigpa* that frame many of the *nang pé men* clinical practices and diagnoses. Within the pulsing of blood are the qualities of the three humours. Imbalance in these three forces and subsequent illnesses are identified in the discrepancies of pulse. For example, as Dönden explains, 'A bile pulse is thin and taut. The phlegm pulse beat is sunken and declining' (1986: 95). Imbalanced humours and the particular beat of the pulse in different locations will indicate to the *drungtsho* what type of disorder the patient might have. However, pulse reading gets far more complex than simply observing three humours; much

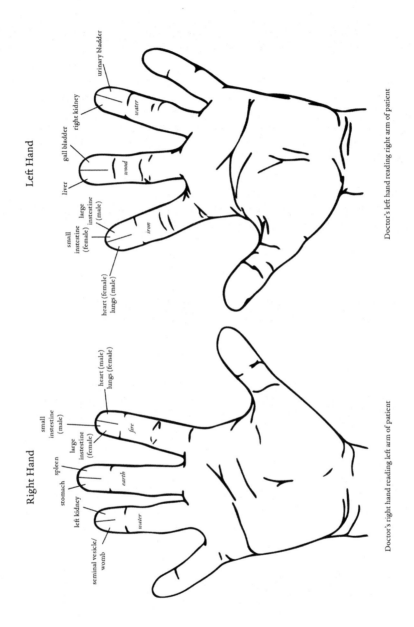

Figure 2.3 A *Drungtsho*'s Hands and Fingertips for Pulse Reading; Drungtsho hands showing the fingertips used to identify specific organ and element pulses. Source: Dönden (1986: 90). From *Health through Balance: An Introduction to Tibetan Medicine* by Yeshi Donden, edited and translated by Jeffrey Hopkins, © 1986 by Dr. Yeshi Dunden. Reprinted by arrangement with The Permissions Company, Inc., on behalf of Shambhala Publications Inc., www.shambhala.com.

more information can be ascertained by the finger positions of the pulse reader, the time of reading, the number of beats during respiratory cycles, the patient diet, finger pressure and patient constitution. This latter factor involves the balance of the patient's five elements – water, earth, fire, iron and wood – all of which can be specific to individual patients. Taking these variables into account, *drungtsho* use the tactile pulse readings to identify disorder types and the quality of internal organ functions (see figure 2.3 depicting fingertip locations and organ identification). Pulse reading is embedded in Buddhist cosmology and philosophy, so it can also be used, along with identifying illnesses, as a type of divination, providing insight into real-life outcomes to family, friends and enemies (Dönden 1986: 85). It can detect the malevolent activities of spirits that can cause illness (88–89) as well as troubled relations with deities. It can also predict life spans, death events and pregnancies, all of which fit into the Buddhist wheel of life.

In the approximately four hundred traditional medicine consultations that I observed, effort and concentration towards this tactile diagnostic technique varied. Often the *drungtsho* stopped talking, followed by the silence of all others in the room. They dipped their heads slightly, as though they were straining to hear something 'in' the patient. However, focus may have been cast elsewhere, such as to a conversation, a telephone call or another distraction. I witnessed one pulse reading where the *drungtsho* paused the reading to answer a call on his mobile telephone, talking briskly while he continued to grip the wrist. The length of time to take a pulse may also vary, with some occurring in less than ten seconds while more diligent readings may take up to a minute or longer. It is difficult to say if this variance in focus undermines the accuracy of the pulse reading; it is quite possible that a pulse can be read with the interjection of a telephone call. The test is a tactile practice that works on sliding scales of phenomenological intensity, not on numeric determinants or conclusive binaries. Thus the medical phenomenology is cumulative, intertwined with many other qualitative markers of examination such as questioning and urine analysis. Those that teach the art of pulse reading say that it takes years to perfect, and repeated practice is necessary to slowly increase a *drungtsho*'s ability to discover the subtleties embedded in the beats. From the *drungtsho*'s perspective, who may read up to fifty different pulses a day, lapse in focus for a few of these analyses may not deduct from their increase in ability over time, especially when the questioning of a patient has revealed the suspected cause of illness. From the patient's perspective, there is little to no outcry over a seemingly lackadaisical pulse reading.

This examination technique is at the heart of the romanticism and allure of Bhutan's traditional medicine. Pulse reading embodies a convergence of cosmology, religion and flesh – on each beat the *drungtsho* feels a patient's wrist, skin, vein, pulse, humours, elements, spiritual being, karma, Samsāric position and environmental history. Because of this convergence, pictures of pulse reading often crop up on publications discussing or exemplifying the *nang pé*

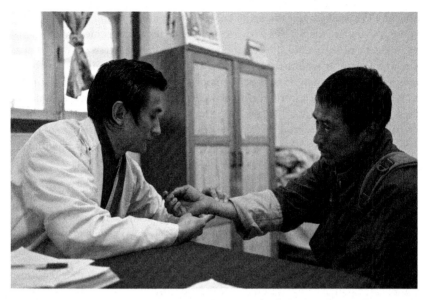

Illustration 2.3 Pulse Reading, *Lhuntse Hospital, Lhuntse*. A *drungtsho* recently graduated from the Faculty of Traditional Medicine reads the pulse of a patient.

men practice, including newspapers, ministry presentations and institutional reports. The iconic and representational image of pulse reading highlights how the practice extends beyond its biomedical counterpart into a more spiritual-religious dimension of body and health.

But pulse reading goes beyond iconic imagery. It plays an important role in the becoming of a patient within a *nang pé men* epistemology and institution. While many patients do not understand the theory of *sowa rigpa*, pulse reading is one of the best-known activities of the practice. It's common to see patients requesting a pulse reading, preemptively pulling up their sleeves, offering their wrists, even if the *drungtsho* does not require it. A *drungtsho* told me that one reason why he performs pulse readings is so that patients feel 'seen'. The physical touch carries an assumed communication of health from patient to *drungtsho*, an offering patients are keen to give during a consultation, with little concern for diagnostic efficacy. In doing so, patients are choosing to enact their bodies within the *nang pé men* epistemology. The results of these tests are written on the patient record sheet, transferring body knowledge to text, cementing this enactment in referential materials that go on to effect the treatment courses and possibilities for referral. Ultimately this popular exchange – the interaction between patient, health institution and medial knowledge – is a process of becoming a bio-traditional citizen.

Once the pulse has been read, there may be a few more questions, a tongue examination, or a urine analysis; however, the latter is rare. On the occasions I did see a *drungtsho* request a urine analysis, the patient would have to return home and prepare themselves with a sample. If a patient had come that day with a sample, he or she would subtly hand it to the *drungtsho*, often concealed in a disposable bag. It would then be taken to a separate room in the hospital reserved for urine analysis where the colour, temperature, vapour and albumin, a cloud-like substance in the urine, would be examined. Like pulse analysis, these properties indicate the balance of the patient's humours, their elemental constitution and potential diseases. Urine analysis is particularly useful for differentiating between hot and cold disorders, a branching of specific illness types within the *sowa rigpa* canon. As Dönden (1986: 122) explains,

> When a heat disorder is present, the urine will be either red or yellow, and it will tend to be rather thick with a foul odour and have a great deal of vapour which lasts a long time. The bubbles that rise to the surface will be small, many, and quickly vanish, and the oily chyle that rises to the surface will be in a thick layer. The albumin will pervade the entire urine, tending to converse towards the centre of the vessel.

I did not see many instances of urine examination in the hospital. It requires complicated patient preparation. Certain foods and liquids as well as vigorous exercise must be avoided before a sample is taken. The sample must also be collected around dawn, with the first half of the urine discarded (for more details on *sowa rigpa* urine analysis see Dönden 1986: 113–30). Such practical complications and delicate handling of the testing makes it a challenging endeavour for both patient and *drungtsho* to gain accurate and effective results. Both the patient and *drungtsho* must be committed to a level of coaching and preparation. Thus urine analysis is typically used for returning patients suffering from chronic or undiagnosed illnesses that have been under the care of a single *drungtsho* for some time.

A complicated testing procedure like urine analysis is another way that patients are presenting their bodies to the *nang pé men* services for amelioration and, in turn, enacting this *nang pé men* conception of health and illness. As I will show in the next section, these enactments of a practice are starting to change the way both patients and the nation-state think about and conceive of healthiness and healing. Due to the institutionalization and nationalization of these processes and the *nang pé men* ethics that are emerging in its wake, I will argue that these new forms of patient are constitutive of a bio-traditional citizenship.

New Bio-traditional Citizens:
Diagnosis, Ethics and an Emerging Traditional Body

As the institution of traditional medicine grows and affects patients within its epistemological and practice bounds, new formations of ethics, bodies and health are emerging. The ethnography of this chapter has shown some of the ways in which the institution of *nang pé men* interacts with its patients through consultations and a network of national clinics. I now wish to turn to one specific dimension of this interaction to demonstrate the complexity and productivity of new forms of medical knowledge both within an institution and to the patients it serves: the diagnosis.

With all examinations finished the *drungtsho* attempts a diagnosis. This is done by applying the results of the diagnostic procedures to the qualities of the 404 *nang pé men* disorders, which are interlinked with the three humours. *Nang pé men* has a large diagnostic directory; *sowa rigpa* uses a disease-classification system related to many different health-influencing variables, such as environmental factors, disorder locations in the body, humour types and even astrology and social contexts. There are 101 disorders influenced by karmic action in previous lifetimes, 101 disorders of this lifetime, 101 disorders caused by spirits or ghosts and 101 'superficial' disorders (see Dönden 1986 and 2000 for more details). The latter includes dietary habits, behaviour patterns, and environmental and social factors. For example, there is a big difference between a patient who visits a *drungtsho* in their hometown in the summer with the support of their family and a patient who is travelling in a foreign environment, differing altitudes and climate, in the winter, alone. Situational specificity is a key part of the diagnosis, and the medicines prescribed will reflect these determining particulars.

A diagnosis, an informed estimation of an illness and an implied cause, is a 'social body' assemblage derived from medical knowledge and the social context in which it is formed. It exists in the social space between a patient, *drungtsho* and a healing practice's epistemology, and it is applied to the patient's body, person and material records. Biomedicine has built firm ethical practices surrounding the disclosure of diagnoses to patients and other third parties (see Reig and Gracia 1992 and Post 2000). While biomedical communities may have differing rules to govern the ethics of disclosure, patients have the right to know their diagnosis, and it is common practice for physicians to explain it to them. In many societies where biomedicine has proliferated as the dominant medical practice, patients are often eager to discover their diagnosis, a shared social body knowledge, which can then be leveraged to access particular treatments and services. Petryna (2008) demonstrates such uses of biomedical identity in her ethnography of the aftermath of the Chernobyl disaster where specific biomedical diagnoses and corresponding patient records offered access to state healthcare resources. In this case, patients were very aware of these diagnoses and their value for healthcare accessibility.

Diagnostic disclosure in Bhutan's *nang pé men* practice varies greatly from the ethical imperatives set out by biomedicine. At the conclusion of a *nang pé men* consultation, *drungtsho* often do not tell the patient their diagnosis, nor do they explain the medical theory behind it. Most patients will leave with a prescription for medicines or therapy but without a firm understanding of the disease or illness that afflicts them. This is not always the case; some diligent patients will extract or communicative *drungtsho* will yield a diagnosis and explanation. In most cases where a diagnosis is given, it is often intimated as a humoural imbalance. For example, a patient might be told they have a wind, bile or phlegm disorder. However, further details into the subsets of these disorders can be scarce, as are wider explanations about *nang pé men* theory.

Overall, there is little institutional imperative to declare diagnostic information, and it is up to the persuasiveness and diligence of the individuals in the consultation to arrive at a shared diagnostic conclusion. Given the enactment of respect by the patient, the position and status of power inhabited by the *drungtsho*, and a general lack of education surrounding *sowa rigpa*, such a conclusion is rare.

While patients of biomedicine are often aware of and searching for a diagnosis, patients of *nang pé men* seem content in not knowing. For the *drungtsho* there is little ethical obligation to deliver a diagnosis. Patients have concern for their welfare and healthiness, and will 'work' in a consultation towards this amelioration by demanding medicines or therapy, but this rarely includes the receipt of a categorical diagnosis. Take for example the following conversation between a *drungtsho* and patient suffering from lower back pain. The *drungtsho* presses for diagnostic questioning, specifically exploring a suspected symptom, while the patient ignores these questions and asks for medicines. For the patient, the medication is the goal, not the diagnosis,

DRUNGTSHO: Are there abnormalities when peeing?
PATIENT: Everything is fine.
DRUNGTSHO: Okay.
[A slight pause]
PATIENT: Aren't you going to give me medicines?
DRUNGTSHO: Sure, you are getting medicines, but you are taking the medicines prescribed by the general hospital?
PATIENT: Yes, but the medicines are all 'Ayurvedic' and I can take along with yours, right?
DRUNGTSHO: Yeah you can take. But when are you are taking the medicines, before or after food?
PATIENT: I am taking three medicines before food.
[A pause]
DRUNGTSHO: Aren't there abnormalities when peeing?
PATIENT: The medicines you provide, will I have to take after food and keep a half hour gap?
DRUNGTSHO: Aren't there abnormalities when peeing?
PATIENT: Half an hour before or after food?
DRUNGTSHO: You are eating the other medicines before food but the medicines from here should be taken half an hour after food. If you are taking the other medicines after food then you should take these medicines before food. Understood?
PATIENT: Yes.

This is a typical conversation in a *drungtsho* office, where the patient seeks to gain and understand an amelioration technique, either in medication, therapy or referral, but does not concern themselves with the diagnosis. In this example, the patient is concerned with how to manage the treatment, in this case medication. The *drungtsho* is attempting to ask diagnostic questions. Eventually he relents to the patient's persistence and explains the medications, leaving the diagnosis undiscussed and only written on the record sheet.

How this diagnosis is written provides an important window into an emerging diagnostic disclosure ethic within traditional medicine. Without a large demand by patients to know a diagnosis, the institution of *nang pé men* is for now happy to provide what the patient wants. Furthermore, the ethical absence of diagnostic disclosure has been internalized by the *nang pé men* institution, in that diagnoses have been concealed and obfuscated from patients by a disease-coding system.

In 2009, with the support of the World Health Organization, the National Traditional Medicine Hospital created the Traditional Medicine Disease Classification (NTMH 2011). Now in its second edition, written only in Dzongkha, bound in a thick green cover, this book sits on *drungtsho* desks all around the county. Every disease type in the *nang pé men* canon has been coded and defined using a simple alphabetic and numerical counting structure. For example, disease 'ka ka 09' (*ka* being the first letter of the Dzongkha alphabet) relates to leg pain, accompanied by redness, burning and/or numbness, which is caused by an agitation of the phlegm and wind humours. The book is extensive and in-depth, an attempt to align with the World Health Organization's International Disease Classification (IDC) system that codes and defines biomedical diseases, making possible international cross-referencing. The World Health Organization extended the IDC to traditional medicines with the International Classification of Traditional Medicine project, launched in December 2010. As the press release for the new project described,

> Several countries have created national standards for the classification of traditional medicine but there is no international platform that allows the harmonization of data for clinical, epidemiological and statistical use. There is a need for this information to allow clinicians, researchers and policy-makers to comprehensively monitor safety, efficacy, use, spending and trends in health care. . . . The classification will initially focus on traditional medicine practices from China, Japan and the Republic of Korea that have evolved and spread worldwide.

The National Traditional Medicine Hospital was interested in this international standardization effort and discussed participation with the World Health Organization's office in Thimphu. Although immediate entry to the project was not recommended due to the absence of a pre-existing codification resource for *nang pé men* diseases in Bhutan, the National Traditional Medicine Hospital has worked for two years to create the classification. The hospital hopes to extend this project into the international efforts of the World Health Organization, and in doing so it aims to open itself to potential funding streams, international recognition and cross-medicine dialogue. As of June 2012 the hospital has begun rolling out this codification project into its patient-management system, with plans to expand it in the future.

Back in the consultation room of the traditional hospital, when *drungtsho* are ready to diagnose the illness, they write a code, perhaps '*ka ka 09*', on the patient record sheet within a field labelled 'disease code' (*nad gzhi'i ang rtags*). The 404 disease codes are too numerous to memorize, especially considering *drungtsho* have already committed to memory the four thick *sowa rigpa* textbooks as part of their training. Twenty or so of the most common diseases are listed on a laminated 'fly sheet' that accompanies the green books, making the referencing process quicker.

When the *drungtsho* returns the yellow patient record sheet with the prescriptions on it, along with instructions for when and how to take the medication, the diagnosis is obfuscated by this disease code, unreadable to anyone without the Traditional Medicine Disease Classification.

I sat in two different *drungtsho* consultation rooms in different parts of the country and asked the same question: When you write the disease code, does the patient know what the diagnosis is? The answers were similar: 'No, and it's better that way.' They explained that they used to write the disease name and explanation before they had the codes, but this caused problems. The patients would sometimes challenge them about the diagnosis. For example, they told me how monks who have knowledge of *nang pé men* might see the diagnosis and complain that they were giving a 'hot' medicine for a 'cold' disorder. The *drungtsho* complained that such patients think they know better than them. They also thought it was easier if the patient didn't know the diagnosis; it was complicated to explain *nang pé men* to the patients, and too much information might even scare them.

The argument set forth by these two *drungtsho* exemplifies the different ethics defining the disclosure of medical knowledge. It also demonstrates the interplay of power in the assembling of bio-traditional citizens between the institution and its patients. Baked into the patient management system itself, on a record sheet that the patient maintains in their possession before and after a consultation, is a restrictor of body knowledge, a code, a textual concealment. However, this is not taken as a negative institutional development by the patient or administrative staff. Without the right to know one's diagnosis, there is little to no complaint from the patient. Rather, with the binding principle to best treat the patient, the moral imperative is reversed: it is best to hide information that is deemed extraneous and potentially damaging from the patient to aid healing. This ethic guides and sustains diagnostic concealment.

Who then uses this coded information and what 'work' does it do for the institution of *nang pé men*? On 1 July 2012 computers were turned on in dispensaries across the country. Each patient that visited a dispensary had their disease codes inputted into a Dzongkha medical database, along with the medicines prescribed. After using this system for some time, a new data set will be available for the National Traditional Medicine Hospital, one that will evidence the types of *nang pé men* diseases afflicting the nation's patients, as well as trends between years, seasons, geography, ages, sexes, income groups, urban and rural populations, among others. An example of a result might read '68% of all female patients seen by the National Traditional Medicine Hospital suffered from wind (*lung*) disorders.' This new data set will sit alongside national health indicators such as 'Diabetes Incidence', 'Conjunctivitis Incidence' or 'Depression Incidence' (MoH 2012a: 17). The latter biomedical illness indicates an agitated wind (*lung*) humour; the possibilities for cross-referencing of data sets are evident. With this new institutional codification venture, the hospital stands on the verge of better inserting itself into national health policy and reporting, and perhaps even meeting some of the efficacy and transparency demands discussed earlier.

This new information system marks a bifurcation in the institute's expansion activities. On the one hand, the hospital is producing a new type of medical knowledge, one that defines the body and health within a *nang pé men* framework, and might offer new and useful ways to monitor and analyze national health trends. But on the other hand, it is reducing the potential of this knowledge to spread among its patients through diagnostic concealment and the lack of public outreach.

This bifurcation poses a threat to the sustainability of the institution of *nang pé men* in Bhutan. Without a clear proliferation of *nang pé men* diagnoses, the medical body is left to be defined by biomedicine. An example of this is the encroachment of biomedical diagnoses in the *nang pé men* hospital. Diagnoses like diabetes are used by *drungtsho* regularly. A *nang pé men* equivalent is available, but for the sake of inter-medicine communication and popular understanding, the biomedical term supersedes. An informal debate is underway between doctors and *drungtsho* about whether *nang pé men* can be used to treat diabetes, meanwhile patients seek traditional medications to stabilize blood sugar levels without the means to measure it. Much can be unpacked from this debate; however, the point here is to show how the biomedical definitions of the body and its medical understanding, in this case 'blood sugar levels' and its relation to the pancreas, have entered the *nang pé men* terminology and practice. While cross-pollination between practices is a shoo-in (two institutional practices that share the same patients and overseeing ministry are sure to exchange medical knowledge), there is mounting concern among *drungtsho* that the exchange of knowledge is predominantly one way and that biomedicine will eventually territorialize the political, epistemological and practice levels of medicine in Bhutan. A good example of this complaint is that English biomedical terms are used in the *nang pé men* hospitals and clinics nationwide, but never did I hear a Dzongkha *nang pé men* term used in the wards and consultation offices of the biomedical hospitals.

While *nang pé men* services are working towards a diagnostic concealment, the biomedical services of Bhutan are working in the opposite direction.

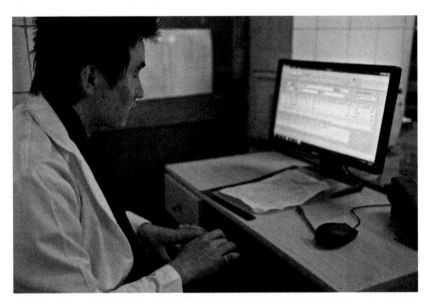

Illustration 2.4 Tracking Traditional-Medicine (2.7, JT 2.7) Patients and Diseases, *National Traditional Medicine Hospital, Thimphu.* A *menpa* in the dispensary inputs patient details, disease codes and prescribed medicines into a database.

Disease categories and nomenclature are pushed onto patients in numerous settings and ways, including consultations and public health programming. For example, the English terms HIV, diabetes, antibiotics, liver disease, obesity and cancer are now commonplace among many Bhutanese patients (see MoH 2008b for a history of HIV in Bhutan). Doctors will use these terms in consultations to explain illness, and patients will in turn use these terms to self-describe illnesses. However, characteristics of their comprehension are questionable, and many doctors say that patients do not understand what a disease like 'cancer' really is, in the biomedical definition. Doctors are in a constant state of persuasive argument with patients. In consultations and hospital rounds doctors are trying to explain the diagnosis and its implications. These efforts are affecting patient medical knowledge on a national scale. Biomedical interpretations of diseases are spreading. On a popular Bhutan Broadcast Service evening show called *Doctors Questions*, many Bhutanese call in to a doctor who answers medical-related questions live. The breadth of questions is vast, with people voicing concerns regarding tumours, cancers, sexually transmitted diseases and much more. The knowledge and deployment of biomedical categories of illness, as well as the accompaniment of assembling biological citizens, is increasing yearly.

Conclusion: Bio-traditional Citizenship

Expanding Petryna's (2002) theory of biological citizenship to include a *nang pé men* dimension is useful in interpreting the proliferation or stagnation of traditional-medicine knowledge across all forms of government, institutions and the public sphere. It is clear from the ways that the *nang pé men* institution interacts with its patients through consultations and its national clinic network that it is attempting to redefine the 'patient' and their 'health' within its own medical knowledge. Given that this medical service operates on a national scale and is supported both financially and politically by the state, therefore identifying patient-citizens within its institutional purview, it is thus pushing forward a new form of bio-traditional citizenship unique to the socio-political contexts of Bhutan.

In turn, patients are slowly beginning to self-identify with this new form of bio-traditional citizenship, using its classifications of body, health and illness to interpret their own experiences of suffering and healing. Pema from chapter 1 is a good case in point: we saw her redefine her nasal illness in the knowledge and practices of *sowa rigpa* after rejecting those of biomedicine. In doing so, she created a new patient multiple and, from the perspective of the National Traditional Medicine Hospital, a new bio-traditional patient case within their institution of care. Through processes of practice enactment, including diagnosis, patient recording and treatment, this new patient-institution relationship, in accordance with the institution's state mandate, was constructive of a bio-traditional citizenship with which patients are able to repeatedly access the state-operated traditional-medicine services. As we learnt about the recent developments in the computational tracking of patient records, such bio-traditional citizenship and its *sowa rigpa* parameters may soon offer the state new ways of conceptualizing the health of its citizens, a 'health' very different from that of the biomedical or biological citizen.

This brings up the challenging institutional relationship between biomedical and traditional services, both of which are agents of citizen-creation. Although *nang pé men* sometimes conceals its diagnostic results from patients, it recognizes the need to face the expansion of biomedical knowledge amongst the population and to add its own epistemological agenda. One recent example of new efforts to further nationalize its practice arrived on televisions across the country; the first *Drungtsho Questions* broadcast live in March 2012. But the uptake is slow and often haphazard; the request for a *drungtsho* to appear on the show came from the Bhutan Broadcast Service, not the hospital, two hours before he was to go live. Institutional expansion activities are ultimately difficult to organize, especially when administrative staff are clinically trained in *nang pé men* and not in hospital management; varying intensities of effort and effectiveness are a constant. The bifurcation in the deployment of diagnostic data between statistical and patient education is one example explored here.

The question for administrators moving forward will be, how does *nang pé men* merge with the biomedical institution and epistemology while maintaining its own identity and substance? In other words, how will the biological and bio-traditional citizenship relate to one another? This is again another example of where the theory of a patient multiple helps to examine how a single person may have two forms of citizenship functioning within the state healthcare services. However, this theoretical approach will still leave questions unanswered on the practical solutions to practice integration. Bhutan's Ministry of Health, the National Traditional Medicine Hospital and their partners will have to find practical ways to achieve constructive integration through policy, institutional structuring, funding and partnered growth (e.g., P. Wangchuk et al. 2007). But these 'big-piece' moves can often either miss the nuances of identity and traditional medicine agency or whitewash it with promises of 'integrative health services'. As the proponents of traditional medicine in Bhutan work out answers to these big questions, they must keep in mind who will be aware of a traditional medicine identity and how: patients, *drungtsho*, or the Ministry of Health? Such questions offer ample areas for further research and institutional development.

While this chapter has explored the efforts of the traditional-medicine institution to create new bio-traditional citizens, one important dimension of this process yet to be discussed is the agency of the patient to partake in or reject this healing option. Patients have the choice whether or not to use the *nang pé men* services, biomedical hospitals or alternative practice, and this position of

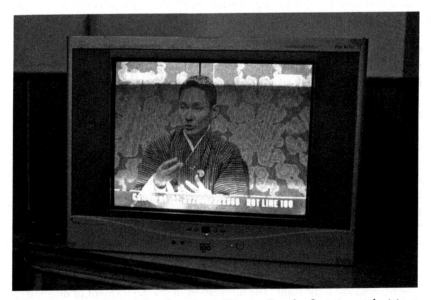

Illustration 2.5 Drungtsho Questions, *Mongar.* For the first time, televisions across Bhutan showed a *drungtsho* fielding questions from the public about health and traditional-medicine's approach to illness and healing.

choice plays a crucial role in patients' experiences, as well as in the institutions' and healers' tactics to attract patients. Chapter 3 will explore the dynamics of this choice and how some of the institutional activities discussed here go on to affect patient decision-making.

Notes

1. The literal translation of *nang pé men* is 'Buddhist medicine', with *nang pé* meaning 'Buddhist'. However, traditional medicine services were seldom referred to as Buddhist medicine, but rather 'traditional medicine' in English translations, such as in the formal institutional name 'National Traditional Medicine Hospital', known in Dzongkha as Gyel Yong (National) Nang Pé (Buddhist) Men Khang (Hospital) Tewa (Centre) (rgyal yongs nang pa'i sman khang lte ba).
2. See the introductory chapter.
3. See Craig 2007 for more on *sowa rigpa* education in Nepal and Tibet.
4. See NTMH 2007 for a standardization guide.
5. Detailed research or publication on the Bhutanese training of drungtsho, menpa and administrative staff is lacking. Much work has been done on the training colleges and methods in Tibet and Nepal (see e.g. Craig 2007a), demonstrating how such curricula and institutional education both fits into and shapes the knowledge and practice of sowa rigpa. Similar research in Bhutan, beyond the scope of this book, is needed to see how similar processes are occurring in the Bhutan context, as well as how biomedicine is worked into the training.
6. See Meyer 1981, 1990 and 1997; Dönden 1986: 75–105; and Gerke 2011: 138–65.

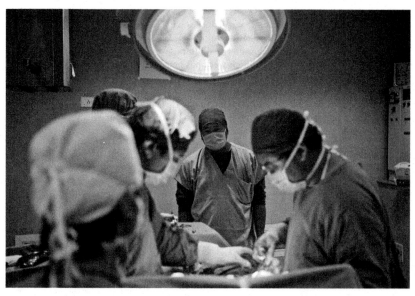

Illustration 3.1 Traditional and Biomedical Integration, *Operation Theatre Two, Mongar Hospital.* In the middle of the photograph stands a traditional medicine *drungtsho.* He was invited by the obstetrics and gynaecology surgeon to witness a caesarean section operation.

3

An Ethnography of Decision-Making

Introducing Some Problems with Healthcare Choice

In the summer of 2011, somewhere in the Haa *dzongkhag*, western Bhutan, high up on a forested mountainside, a woman fell ill. She visited the Haa Hospital where, like all other hospitals across the country, she was presented with a choice, 'Would you like the modern or traditional medicine?' asked the receptionist. She decided to first try the state offering of traditional medicine. She was offered a consultation and a course of traditional medicine. Given the severity of the case, the *drungtsho* instructed the patient to return to the hospital within the week for a follow-up. Sadly, the patient did not return. Two weeks later she was delivered to hospital by ambulance. Her body was completely swollen and her vital signs were weak. She died within a few hours. The biomedical doctor of the hospital who also related the same story told me it had been an autoimmune disease, yet the diagnosis was unknown. Given that there are no autopsy services in Bhutan, we would never find out if he was right. In his office, two doors down from the *drungtsho*'s chamber, he whispered to me that had the patient seen him first he might have been able to help. It wasn't the *drungtsho*'s fault; after all, the *drungtsho*'s job is to cure people, and that is what they tried to do, with good follow-up instructions. The doctor was sensitive and respectful of traditional medicine, as so many of his biomedical colleagues were in Bhutan. The ethic of patient-responsibility is supported by the lack of a formal referral system between biomedical and traditional practices, and, as a result, impetus for crossover between practices is often left with the patient. The doctor paused and looked concerned, then said, 'If only the patient had decided differently, she may have survived.'

At the onset of sickness, patients in Bhutan are presented with a series of healthcare options. Biomedical, traditional or alternative practices offer an assortment of 'choices', strategies and technologies of healing and care that may ameliorate illness. This diversity of choice was institutionalized into two state services offered side by side in national hospitals and clinics, an operational emblem of the Ministry of Health's policy of 'medical integration'. Outside of hospitals, patients engage a huge diversity of healers and alternative practices to complement their healing. The desire to alleviate pain and suffering drives patients to access these choices and eventually make a decision about which practice to use and when. Such decisions can have important repercussions for patients, their families and their communities, and are often critical moments in people's lives. Patients must act on cultural, economic and spiritual beliefs and then manage the consequences to their health.

While the decisions themselves may have a profound effect on patients and their healthiness, the availability of practice choice also plays an important role. As these plural practices continue to grow within the modernizing state of Bhutan, carving out cultural, economic and popular space amongst socialities of healing, a new ethics of 'appropriate practice' is emerging. Biomedical, traditional and alternative practitioners are engaging patients within these emerging ethics, arguing for or against particular healthcare choices. Thus both the availability of choice and the ethics that organize and arrange these choices are having a new and profound effect on patients.

The aim of this chapter is to examine how the availability of plural healthcare choice and resultant processes of decision-making affects patients. Specifically it will look at some of the repercussions of choice between practices and what happens when decisions are made. Given the critical nature of some of these decisions, the question of effective or appropriate care arises both for patients and health practitioners. So by exploring choice and decision-making, this chapter examines the ethics of what is 'effective care'.

The first section of this chapter explores the complexity of choices within healthcare decision-making processes and looks at some of the factors influencing patients and their families. It investigates the ethnographic narrative of Tshomo and Sonam, two new parents deciding whether to visit the Mongar biomedical hospital unit or conduct a religious healing ritual with their village *lama*, or both, for the treatment of their one-day-old newborn who was unable to feed. The decision was critical as the baby was dehydrated, jaundiced and close to death. Ultimately the parents decided to visit the hospital and the baby survived through rapid attention in the intensive care unit. Meanwhile they also conducted the religious ritual at home. The deliberation to visit hospital exemplifies the dangers of having diverse healthcare options and the challenges of matching certain types of healthcare knowledge to appropriate treatment routes.

The final section expands on the issues of 'appropriate care' as it plays out in the social, political and multi-medical contexts of Bhutan. While patients straddle differing practitioners and medical knowledge, they also assemble divergent aetiological epistemologies, locating the sources of illness and disease in differing subjects. My work has found that with the onus on the patient to decide when and where to seek medical help, beliefs surrounding causation are tantamount to 'first-response' behaviours. A second ethnographic example involves Dechen, a three-year-old girl, suffering from acute pain in her left arm. The story details how the parents preferred *rim dro* and shamanic treatments in the first four months of the disease due to aetiological beliefs involving the socio-religious exchanges between a mountain deity and the villagers. On arrival to hospital, the biomedical and traditional doctors voiced outrage at the delay in seeking appropriate treatment and the resultant worsening of what was finally diagnosed as 'osteomyelitis'. Instances of delayed hospital visitation are a common complaint from biomedical and traditional doctors, and such delay is an active point of reform within the Ministry of Health's public health agenda. These two differing perspectives on causation of disease and the resultant persuasion tactics deployed by different interlocutors play out in many of the health spheres in Bhutan, including politics, media and religious institutions, instances of which are described in conjunction with this case. As a result, practices and health epistemologies are being defined, delineated and disputed, with conceptions of 'appropriate care' changing in the wake of such debates.

One important outcome from these two ethnographic narratives is that patients seldom select between practices, either alternative or biomedical. In the everyday reality of decision-making processes, patients are rarely troubled by or rejective of mutually exclusive views of practices, healths and bodies. They would rather use practices and conceptions of health and illness causation in tandem and in complement with one another. Variations of practices, healths and bodies would amalgamate in a continuum of healing assemblages, and are available to the patient to use as and when they seek care. As further described in the conclusion of this book, patients' experiences of healing and suffering are thus formed more by the organization, management and performing of differing healthcare choices, as in which one to use first or in which order, rather than in the selection and rejection of certain practices.

I conclude that while alternative practices are still being used, typically in tandem with state health services (albeit for divergent epistemological reasons), the knowledge and healthcare-seeking behaviour of many Bhutanese is changing rapidly. Clearly the proactive and enlightened approach of the Bhutanese government since the early 1900s has thus far protected alternative practices and beliefs, encouraging medical diversity. However, as ideas of health and appropriate care are increasingly territorialized by institutional health agendas, the future of practice diversity becomes questionable, even more so when human lives and their sufferings are more rigorously accounted for by media coverage, legislation, health statistics and monitoring programmes. Patients are demanding more from both state services and alternative practitioners. Meanwhile the Ministry of Health is requesting that all alternative practitioners register under the Bhutan Medical and Health Council, a tall order for many who fear punitive responses to their practices. Ultimately alternative practitioners increasingly have to defend their effectiveness and applicability to a changing patient understanding of health and what is or what is not an appropriate treatment. The next decade of health policy, patient decision-making and practitioner accountability will play a key role in deciding what will happen to Bhutan's diverse medical pluralism.

Before proceeding, I want to make a distinction between 'choice' and 'decision'. For the clarity and purpose of this chapter, I use the term 'choice' to refer to the plural healthcare options available to patients, introduced in chapter 1. 'Choice' describes an array of options, potential treatment routes, available, waiting, open. An example could be, 'When Dorji fell ill, he had many choices of practices, and he wasn't sure which one to use.' I will never use this term as a verb to describe 'choosing' between practices. The term 'decision' will be used in these instances. For example, 'Dorji had a wide variety of choices, but finally made the decision to use his village *lama*.' 'Decisions' are active selections between 'choices'.

The Criticality of a Newborn

In the winter of 2011, Sonam and Tshomo were happily expecting their first child. They had prepared, both knowingly and unknowingly, for the past thirty years for this moment. They had fallen in love in Trashigang four years after completing their teacher training college in Thimphu, where after many years of successful education themselves they had both decided to teach. They had married recently, in their early thirties, a late age that required some rehearsed explaining. Sonam told me that they had both focused on their teaching careers and that is why they both had waited uncommonly long to settle down with a partner. They had been responsible until this point and had not run off to elope, choosing instead the more appropriate and respected strategy of finishing their studies and training before marrying. This way, their careers and livelihoods would be assured before starting a family. Their patience and acumen surrounding their union spoke to a responsible and intricate self-management that was being rewarded by a stable and happy life together. They owned a home in a small village just next to the main road between the east and west of Bhutan, only forty-five minutes from Mongar. The village lies low in the base of a valley surrounded by lush green jungle forests, supported by the hot and humid temperatures of this atypically low-altitude area.

With the civil service now the largest single employer in the country, including the state education system (see Upadhyay 2000), it is common to meet couples in Bhutan who work in government jobs that require remote national postings. I met countless men and woman who were in relationships, engaged or married but lived apart from their partners or children, sometimes not seeing them for months or years. The desire for lucrative and stable yet inconveniently located civil-service jobs has made long-distance relationships commonplace. Suffering in the throes of a long-distance relationship myself, I was constantly amazed at the matter-of-factness with which couples would normalize and manage the prospects of sometimes years apart, perhaps without any concrete guarantees of eventually living together. This is not to say that long-distance woes were absent, but that such personal relationships were common.

Sonam and Tshomo faced these issues, but they were politically and socially savvy enough to arrange a co-placement. The school in their village needed two new teachers, and they negotiated their way to the top of the list together.

Not only did they craftily locate themselves in the same village professionally but they also showed remarkable forethought regarding Tshomo's pregnancy. Like many Bhutanese, they were sexually active before their marriage and after. They used contraception to delay a pregnancy that they both wanted, but not until the right time. After a few years of working and saving, they were ready. They purposely conceived their child in March 2011 so that it would arrive during the December school holiday and that neither parent would miss any work. Even though an element of biological luck was involved in conception, they demonstrated a strong ability to manage their lives in some very challenging external circumstances, including reproductive biology, family livelihood and institutional responsibilities.

Having come from rural farming families, now in their early thirties and benefitting from a stable salary, they represent a booming working class of Bhutanese who have lived and trained in urban centres and returned to rural villages or towns. Urban exposure and rigorous education had left them with a strong understanding of the state healthcare options, both traditional and biomedical. They were well-versed with the Ministry of Health's public health initiative to manage all births in medical clinics, ideally a large hospital with an obstetrics and gynaecology unit, like the one in Mongar Hospital. For those too far from such services, BHUs, including the one in their village, have been kitted out with birthing units, typically staffed by trained health assistants who can aid in births and make immediate referrals when faced with complications. Tshomo was persuaded by her BHU's health assistant to attend regular pre-natal checkups, as well as to give birth in the BHU. Sonam often accompanied her, and he supported her throughout the pregnancy and birth. He had taken on the responsibilities of a supportive father and was prepared when the big day came. Their willingness to participate in biomedical pre-natal and childbirth services was not forced or coerced, language that might be used by some public health workers engaging with rural populations. They were already convinced of the value of biomedical care by their past education and exposure to the state provision. Sonam was particularly appreciative of the public health programming on the Bhutan Broadcast Service, especially the television show *Doctors Questions*. He felt he had learnt a lot about health and treatment from the biomedical doctors answering the public's inquiries. Both parents wanted the help of the biomedical services in pre-natal and labour care.

Their remote posting meant that Sonam and Tshomo were relatively isolated from community and family. They seldom saw their extended family who lived east of Mongar. Like many other civil-service employees, they were relatively unfamiliar with their new community. Moving to a new place can be lonely as language and culture vary drastically between the regions of Bhutan. I saw many lonely single BHU workers who were posted for over three years in what

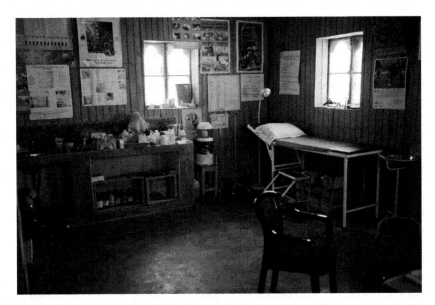

Illustration 3.2. Inside a BHU, *Lingshi Dzongkhag.* The walls are covered with public health posters, some over ten years old. For a rural BHU like this one, staffed by a single health assistant, sick persons are usually asked to come into the health clinic for treatment. Due to the daily patient demand and the lack of staff, health assistants often can't visit patients in their homes.

they considered isolated social settings. While Sonam and Tshomo were lucky to have one another, isolation played an important role in the events post-birth. Without ready access to a community or familial network, they were reliant on the knowledge provided by public health education and their BHU. As many new parents worldwide can probably attest, not even the most rigorous reading and study can fully prepare you for the trials of childbirth and neonatal care. Community expertise, in or out of medical institutions, often provides vital support. Sonam and Tshomo lacked these networks. Possibly they were also overconfident in their own relatively high level of education and public health knowledge. Such educational inequality could have isolated them further, as both they and their less well-educated neighbours could have assumed they had obtained sufficient knowledge. This relative isolation was a compounding factor to what follows.

I met Tshomo and Sonam in the intensive care unit of Mongar Hospital where their newborn son was being treated for what biomedicine describes as dehydration and jaundice. Neonatal jaundice is one of the most common vulnerabilities for newborns, often considered a normal part of the post-birth process (Maisels and Watchko 2000). Approximately 60 percent of term and 80 percent of pre-term infants develop light symptoms within the first week (Tidy

2010; National Institute of Health and Care Excellence 2010). Initial symptoms include a light yellowing of skin, slight stupor or lethargy, paucity of movement and poor sucking (feeding). More severe cases may present increased yellowness, sclera, drowsiness, moderate to deep stupor, minimal feeding, high-pitched crying and changes in muscle tone (Maisels 2005: 768–846), all of which signal a dangerous brain dysfunction called kernicterus, a cause of cerebral palsy (Crigler and Najjar 1952; Maisels 2006: 443). Neonatal jaundice follows hyperbilirubinemia, an elevation of serum bilirubin levels, often linked to blockages of faecal matter in the gut (Maisels 2006: 443–44). For most babies that feed well, these blockages are removed with defecation and the jaundice is relieved within a week. In cases of limited feeding and subsequent dehydration, the blockages can remain, leaking faecal toxins into the gut and further elevating bilirubin levels (445). Babies are particularly vulnerable to neonatal jaundice in the first seventy-two hours after birth because, 'until the milk has "come in," breastfed infants receive fewer calories, and the decrease in caloric intake is an important stimulus to increasing the enterohepatic circulation' (445), which produces bilirubin. The American Academy of Paediatrics recommends that any infant discharged at less than seventy-two hours of age should be seen within two days of discharge, to ensure that the baby is receiving enough milk, defecating and not showing signs of jaundice (447). Biomedical treatment includes ultraviolet phototherapy (Stokowski 2006 and Maisels 2006: 450–52), exchange transfusion (Maisels 2006: 452) and controlled rehydration (Harrison 2008: 365). If neonatal jaundice goes untreated, it can lead to permanent brain damage or death (Crigler and Najjar 1952).

Over the course of a few days as their son was treated with phototherapy and rehydration by the paediatrician, Tshomo, Sonam and I discussed their story at length. Being teachers who were relatively open to the idea of ethnographic research, they were forthcoming about the birth and the days that followed. They told me how Tshomo had given birth successfully in the BHU with the help of the clinic's health assistant, in the supine position with legs suspended in stirrups.[1] The health assistant was trained in delivery but didn't offer sufficient details about neonatal care, specifically about feeding or jaundice. Maisels (2006: 448) lists 'Ten Commandments for Preventing and Managing Hyperbilirubinemia', including the promotion and support for successful breast-feeding, a pre-discharge systematic assessment for hyperbilirubinemia, the provision of jaundice information and early warning signs to parents in case of developing complications, and follow-ups based on the time of discharge. None of these were provided to Sonam and Tshomo for their newborn, increasing the risk of neonatal jaundice.

For Tshomo to attend the BHU for the birth is a mark of radical change in birthing processes in Bhutan. Due to a big public health push in the last decade, deliveries attended by skilled health personnel have skyrocketed from 23.7 percent in 2000 to 81 percent in 2012 (MoH 2013a: 67). More mothers were visiting health clinics to have their babies. The Ministry of Health advocated this change to lower the infant mortality rate (60.5 in 2000 to 47 in 2010, per 1,000 live births, MoH 2013a: 17). Although progress has been made, the relatively high infant mortality rate demonstrates how difficult it is for biomedical services to offer effective birthing and neonatal care in more remote regions with current human resource limitations. As a result, mothers may come to clinics but might not get the best care and advice.

The birth was uncomplicated and their son appeared healthy and responsive. In the evening the happy new parents took their child home. They had not named him; they were waiting for Sonam's brother to consult a renowned *lama* in Sikkim, India, who would select an appropriate name. Sonam kept his mobile phone close to him, eagerly awaiting the name of his son to arrive by text message. At home, Tshomo lay in bed next to the child. For the several days following community members visited, offered gifts, and were served tea and snacks by a now-exhausted Sonam. Birth was a time of celebration, and although Tshomo and the child would remain in their room, separate from the visitors, the small crowd would sit on floor mats and happily discuss the new community member's arrival and other tidbits of social news. But these visitors would offer little neonatal advice or care. Tshomo's sister, who was living with them at the time, was the only additional person on hand to help care for the newborn, his mother and the daily flow of guests.

A major challenge for paediatric doctors in Bhutan is the misconceptions surrounding the feeding of newborns. While baby formula isn't popular because of its cost and unavailability, new parents are eager to introduce water and rice to children younger than six months. One North American paediatrician on a three-year contract in the Jigme Dorji Wangchuck National Referral Hospital advised new parents to feed only breast milk for the first six months. This was hard advice to fathom; rice is a staple food for most Bhutanese, who are keen to supplement their children's diet with rice as early as possible. The paediatrician's experience was backed by a 1995 study by Bohler and Bergström (1995) that found ninety-eight breastfeeding mothers in Eastern Bhutan supplemented feeding with semisolid foods within three months of birth. Adding some ethnographic data to this quantitative study, Wikan and Barth's book *Situation of Children in Bhutan* (2011:50–51) describes some birthing and infant-care practices in rural communities collected in repeated field trips between 1989 and 1999:

> The child is welcomed into the world by being offered a lump of butter. This is repeated before every feeding from anything from 3 to 15 days, and one proud mother with a particularly healthy child claimed to have done so regularly till the child was past two. . . . Customs with regard to supplementary feeding vary. A supplement of butter and rice flour may be introduced as early as the fourth day of life. Rice flour-paste or wheat flour-paste is introduced into the diet quite early, feeding the child with unwashed fingers or from the mother's or other caretaker's mouth.

To dissuade similar feeding practices encountered by the paediatrician, he made it clear that the child would have a lifetime of eating rice, but for the first six months the child needed the nutritional benefits of 100 percent breast milk. This left little room for doubt or miscommunication with parents, who he was likely not to see again. But this is just one paediatrician in a Thimphu office, and while Wikan and Barth's data is over a decade old, most of my health staff interviewees noted a big variance in neonatal care and feeding, with many risky practices still common.

Given Tshomo's education and pre-natal visits to the BHU, she knew the benefits of breastfeeding, and it had been her intent at the outset to breastfeed. However, when things didn't go as planned, indecision and confusion set in, causing her and Sonam to start deliberating on what action to take.

The problem with breastfeeding started when they returned home from the BHU without enough guidance from the health assistant. In the few hours after birth in the BHU, her son latched onto her breast and fed on some colostrum, but it was unclear to Tshomo, as with so many new mothers, how well he fed. On returning home her milk didn't come in, as it sometimes doesn't for many mothers for one or two days. Their son's feeding on the colostrum was slow and often unsuccessful. Within a day he became drowsy and less interested in feeding. Sonam and Tshomo explained it as droopiness, where vigorous kicking and arm movements slowed and weakened. They waited another three days, expecting the milk to come and feeding to improve. Tshomo lifted her child to her breast to encourage feeding, but the infant seemed disinterested. Sonam and Tshomo became distraught with worry. By the end of the third day, now three and a half days since birth, their child was weak and unresponsive – he ceased cooing and seldom kicked. If he cried it was whiny and high pitched. He wasn't defecating and wouldn't feed. Finally, his forehead started to look yellowish in colour, extending slowly down his face and chest. By this time they knew something was very wrong and began discussing their options.

A compounding issue was the relative isolation of Tshomo and Sonam during this time and their lack of access or consultation with third parties who might have taken them to hospital sooner or supported the breastfeeding effort in other ways. Communities around the world have different support mechanisms for neonatal care. For example, experienced elders may help with breastfeeding technique and knowledge; other breastfeeding mothers might step in for a mother waiting for her milk to come in, or family members with an 'outside' perspective might encourage a hospital visit. All these things happen in Bhutan, but were not available to Sonam and Tshomo. They told me that due to their remote teaching placement and disconnection from the community they didn't have much neonatal support. Only Tshomo's younger sister, who was staying with them and assisting with the neonatal care, was available, and she hadn't any experience with childbirth.

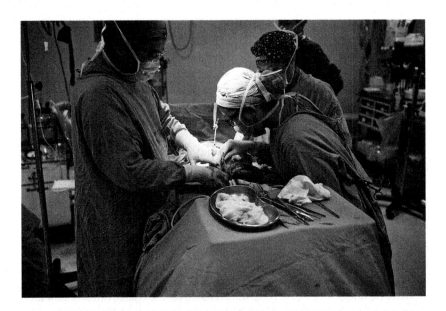

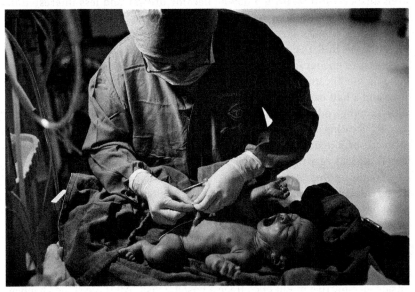

Illustrations 3.3 and 3.4 Birth by Caesarian Section, *Operation Theatre Two, Mongar Hospital.* A baby is pulled from its mother. The surgeon's assistant quickly clears the airway. Within a minute of being born, the baby is whisked to an adjacent room and placed under a heat lamp for post-birth care.

Wikan and Barth confirm this isolation for young mothers in what is some of the only data available on childbirth in Bhutan (2005: 48):

> Our interviews indicate that the majority of women have given birth with assistance only of their husband, unless even he is absent, on work or trade. The topic of childbirth is also little discussed and explained, even among women. As a consequence, knowledge about birth procedures and precautions is poorly distributed, and show great local and individual variation. Thus squatting, on the hands and knees, and grasping a rope suspended from the roof are all reported.

This fieldwork was conducted in the 1990s, before the Ministry of Health's massive push to bring mothers into BHUs for delivery. The isolation during childbirth as noted by Wikan and Barth in conjunction with high infant mortality rates explains the Ministry of Health's efforts to institutionalize the birthing process. While much has changed in the past decade, these findings, along with their remote professional placement away from family, partly explain why Tshomo and Sonam lacked support. Unable to help their child alone, they were going to have to seek healing help.

One choice available to them was to visit Mongar where the hospital's sole paediatrician was available for emergencies and consultations. Sonam had even saved enough money to buy a small car, minimizing the trip to a forty-five minute drive. For many patients needing to visit a hospital, long distances and mountainous topography, as well as the logistics and cost to traverse them, were enough to deter them. But Sonam and Tshomo had vaulted this first hurdle. They knew they had access to this doctor and that it would have been free, bar the cost of fuel. They also knew that this doctor could provide a diagnosis or at least investigate the cause of the child's malaise. The hospital was known to Sonam and Tshomo; they thought very positively of it and valued the effectiveness of biomedicine thus far in their lives. So why did they delay their decision to go to Mongar Hospital?

As their son's symptoms slowly came on over the first few days, one issue within their decision-making process was that they themselves could neither identify the problem nor its cause. Being unable to assess the symptoms, they delayed making a healthcare-seeking decision. In a single-track healthcare situation any malady may be swiftly acted upon by seeking that sole type of treatment. However, in Bhutan's plural-practice context, patients often wait until the source or aetiology of an illness is identified or at least guessed at before seeking care. Their ignorance of possible causes for their child's illness delayed their decision for three days on what type of healing practice would be appropriate.

They were not oblivious to the issues presented on those first two days. They suspected the lack of feeding had something to with their son's worsening malady. They also knew that feeding for newborns could be sporadic and slow at first, with colostrum supporting a child until a mother's milk comes in. However, they had not realized that by day two, without substantial feeding in conjunction with lack of defecation, their son had become dehydrated and jaundiced. When Tshomo's milk came in on day three, the illness had got to a point where the child was no longer able to latch or feed. As her milk became readily available it seemed implausible that the child would not be drinking due to dehydration – there was after all now an ample supply of milk. The mystery surrounding the cause of their child's illness led to speculation that something karmic or spiritual might be afoot. This is when another healthcare treatment choice presented itself.

They contacted the village *lama* and urgently discussed the details of the case. By the end of the third day Sonam and Tshomo were strongly considering conducting a *rim dro* at home to clear any malicious or karmically negative circumstances surrounding the newborn. This ritual would include reciting sacred texts, constructing *torma* (*gtor ma*, small butter statues that act as offerings) and exchanging other gifts from parents to deities in return for karmic balance and spiritual protection. Although these parents had worked hard to assure all the religious aspects of this major life event were adhered to before birth, newborn children are known to be especially susceptible to malevolent spirits, deities and ill-wishers from the community (Wikan and Barth 2005: 47–50). Ritualistic coping strategies are common: for example, it is often considered protective to throw rice away from the front door and house before taking a newborn through the doorway, either in or out. The rice is said to distract any malevolent spirits or ghosts that may be loitering around the property, awaiting the arrival of a child not yet able to protect themselves. Sonam and Tshomo had placed protective items around their son's neck, suspended by blessed necklaces, and had their *lama* conduct a pre-birth ritual. But Sonam and Tshomo came to wonder whether the *lama*'s rite had not sufficiently protected their vulnerable son and whether further religious intervention might alleviate the sufferings of their child and encourage him to feed.

Attitudes towards the treatment of young children by alternative practices are changing. As highlighted in chapter 1's example of Pema using cutting and sucking, there are many other alternative practices besides *rim dro* that engage patients in a more invasive manner. A doctor in the Mongar intensive care unit repeated what I heard from many other doctors, that ten years prior parents would often use these alternative practices on their newborn and young children. He recounted an extreme example where a newborn fell ill and the parents blamed a local deity and its poisoning (*dug*). They opted for the cutting and sucking practice on the child's back, the same practice that Pema used. He recalls seeing the child a few days later, after infection had set in. The child's entire back was engulfed by a putrid wound leaking pus. The surgical specialist at the time had to cut through the wound and drain it, then bandage the entire back. With an intensive course of intravenous antibiotics the child luckily survived but was scarred permanently. After recounting this story, the doctor shrugged and said, 'This was the practice of the time; now people are educated and don't do this.' Although dramatic and infused with a biomedical bias arguing against the use of invasive alternative practices, this story highlights how common these practices were in the recent past. This story is corroborated by further examples of alternative dietary, behavioural and religious practices associated with neonatal care noted by Wikan and Barth (2011: 47–50). Since their 1990s research, there has been a marked reduction in the use of invasive body procedures such as cutting and sucking, burning or moxibustion, in inverse relation to the expansion of biomedical neonatal care and education. During my time in the paediatric units of both Thimphu and Mongar Hospitals, I neither saw nor heard of parents using such invasive methods on their young children. It appears that parents trust the biomedical services to handle acute illnesses if they suspect invasive measures might be needed. But as highlighted in the case of Sonam and Tshomo, while invasive alternative practices are not used on children, non-invasive practices such as a *rim dro* are still very much a part of children's healing narratives, and time taken to conduct such practices can delay the seeking of other types of care.

On the morning of the fourth day, Sonam and Tshomo's son became increasingly unresponsive and lethargic. They had decided to proceed with the religious ritual, and their *lama* was on hand ready to begin a three-day *rim dro*. They were still deliberating on whether to visit Mongar Hospital. Although the decision may appear obvious to some readers, it was not, at the time, obvious to these first-time parents. They genuinely believed that the *rim dro* could be effective, as too could the hospital. If only they could have identified the reason for their child's malady, they would have known exactly what practice to use. But as described in chapter 1, when patients have multiple healths that must be treated in different ways, enforced by multiples of available practices, it becomes challenging to identify, let alone treat, the affected health. The child's rapidly declining state had agitated his parents to the point of indecision. While debate over the appropriate treatment continued, one thing was clear: a decision had to be made about visiting hospital in conjunction with the *rim dro*, and it had to be done that morning.

This highlights a crucial aspect of a patient's decision-making process in contemporary Bhutan: the requirement to manage and assemble responses to illness in the context of the patient multiple. Patients and those who act as decision-makers on their behalf are solely responsible for making their own healthcare decisions amongst the available choices. They hold the agentive power. Although humans are all obviously responsible for their own lives and healthiness, even in less practice-plural contexts, this power must be managed within these decision-making processes. In the case of Sonam and Tshomo, they were considering hospital and alternative treatment. It wasn't so much a decision defined by one practice or another, but rather when and how they should use the practices available. This demonstrates that patients have a complex and challenging task in managing and arranging their patient multiplicity, as well as the practices, healths and bodies that constitute it. This includes identifying illnesses and deciding what is or is not an 'appropriate' treatment type.

Sonam told me that it was Tshomo's younger sister who eventually made the decision for them. She was as educated as the couple and had similar exposure to biomedical and religious healing practices. When she saw that the child was turning yellow in conjunction with the severity of the child's lethargy, she implored them to take the child to hospital immediately. In addition she reasoned that the *lama* could begin the *rim dro* in their absence. Remote *rim dro*, or those performed at home with the home vacant, are not unheard of. In examples where family members persuade patients to visit hospital rather than perform religious ceremonies, these remote *rim dro* are becoming more common, more popular and more acceptable. This rationale of 'best of both worlds' was enough to tip the balance for Sonam and Tshomo. They piled into his tiny car and raced up the winding forested road to Mongar.

By midday Tshomo was resting her arms on a plastic incubator in the intensive care unit of Mongar Hospital, watching over her four-day-old son. He was slowly feeding through a gavange tube and soaking up a lamp's ultraviolet rays through his tiny bare chest. As I stood back and watched her son regain strength, I could hear the sounds of a respirator in the adjacent room; unfortunately those parents had waited too long to visit hospital, and their child had passed away, yet fifteen minutes of small puffs of breath were being maintained as demanded by the intensive care unit's neonatal protocol. Sonam was a few steps away talking with the paediatrician who was softly telling him about dehydration and jaundice in infants. The doctor thought that the boy had been hours away from dying or permanent brain damage. The doctor assured Sonam that his son was going to be okay. Sonam relaxed a little and flipped open his mobile phone to check for his son's name. Meanwhile, back at home, the *lama* was forming small *torma* statues out of coloured butter while reciting mantra, an important and simultaneous practice in the healing of this new young boy.

The inclusion and eventual decisiveness of Tshomo's sister highlights the central role of family and community members within healthcare decision-making processes. While patients are often at the centre of decision-making inquiries in Bhutan, given the level of agency they have in selecting their own care and deciding when to visit a practice, this agency is often dispersed throughout social networks. The locus of decision-making processes is decentred from the patient into wider communities. These communities and how they interpret illness and response are often pivotal in delineating the active ethics of appropriate care by which decisions are made. The following section gives another account of parents who had to make a healthcare-seeking decision on behalf of their ailing child. To do so, they drew upon an ethics of appropriate care that resided in a social and spiritual network linked to their community, geography and religion.

Rupturing and Repairing

Mongar Hospital, constructed between 2005 and 2009 with funding from the Indian government, is a bustling healthcare centre, with doctors, nurses, lab technicians, health assistants, administrative staff, cleaners, maintenance crews, patients and family members in continual motion through its dark halls. Perched just below Mongar town, its large white multi-storey concrete structure dwarfs other buildings in the eastern regions of Bhutan, except for the ancient religious and administrative fortresses known as *dzongs*. Having been positioned on a slope that drops off steeply from the town's main market square and carved into the topography through extensive ground works, the hospital's full spatial presence is hard to comprehend. Strategically placed trees and the dipping horizon of the land make it hard to view the entire edifice at once, allowing only parts of it to be seen and mentally reconstructed as an institutional and structural whole.

Below the main building cascade multiple residences that vary in size and facilities, depending on the occupants' hierarchical ranks in the state medicine system. The hospital's superintendent and full-time biomedical doctors have the pick of the bunch. Proximity housing means that staff are never more than a ten-minute walk from the hospital, although not all staff are lucky enough to acquire free hospital accommodation due to apartment shortages. It also means that the biomedical doctors can be on call twenty-four hours a day, seven days a week, and with only one specialist in each unit, they are frequently called in at all hours of the night.

There is only one place in the Mongar *dzongkhag* where the hospital's mark on the physical landscape can be appreciated: from across the deep valley in the small and dispersed village of Chali. From parts of this adjacent mountainside facing Mongar, the slow sluggish ascent of headlights at night indicate doctors sleepily winding their way back up to the hospital for emergency cases. In daylight the rising white buildings of the hospital's three wings are visible, two of which house the different inpatient wards, the other housing a six-storey sloped gangway allowing gurney access to all floors in case of elevator failure. Although the building looked small to me across the large expanse of the wide valley and I knew it was still over an hour's drive away along a rugged mountain farm road, the hospital was a spectacle, a new mark on the landscape, clearly denoting the advance of healthcare services in a region that not long ago was considered remote and unopened. This distance is both geographical and developmental, with Mongar's infrastructure, demography, culture and economy looking like a metropolis in the agriculturalist community of this small, rural village.[2] Standing in Chali looking across the valley at my fieldsite, I realized that Bhutan doesn't build many new large *dzongs* any more, although they do repair or rebuild them if they burn down (BBS 2012e). Bhutan now builds hospitals that, like Trongsa *dzong* as seen on approach from an adjacent mountainside, rise out of forests and low-lying urban centres to symbolize the eminence, centrality

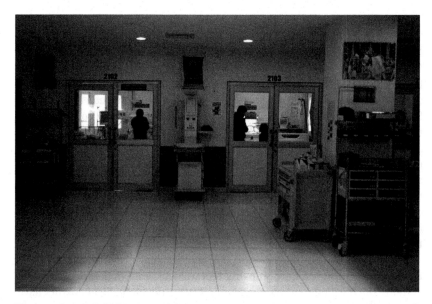

Illustration 3.5 Tshomo and Sonam, *Intensive Care Unit, Mongar Hospital.* Tshomo and Sonam, in the room to the right, stand next to the glowing lights of the phototherapy incubator, watching over their newborn son. In the next room over, a mother grieves.

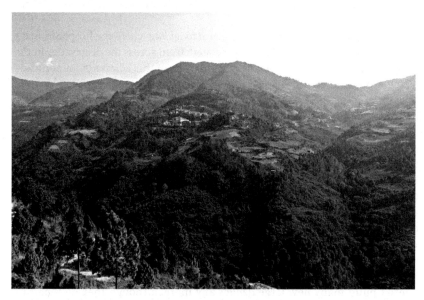

Illustration 3.6 Mongar as Seen from Chali, *Chali, Mongar Dzongkhag.* A view of Mongar Hospital, the large white building across the valley, as seen from the village of Chali.

and power of medical knowledge and practice. Rather than religious and political hegemonies, these recent changes in Bhutan's landscapes are reflective of the shifting socialities of healthcare.

Dechen, a three-year-old girl who sat in the surgical recovery ward of the hospital, was from this small adjacent village of Chali. She was terrified to see me standing at her bedside talking with her parents. I had become better at approaching bedsides tentatively, softly, so as not to shock patients too much. Despite this, I could seldom avoid the stark sit-up and wide-eyed double-takes of patients who didn't expect to see a tall white man in front of them speaking Dzongkha. But Dechen was different. Her response was one of a child worn down by months, possibly years, of pain, a tiredness and physical fatigue that made irritability and forlornness a modus operandi. Yes, it was my difference that scared her, but in her tears and retreat into her mother's arms, she revealed misery that I had come to recognize in some patients who live with chronic pain. Without the hardening of a medical training and long-term exposure to such suffering, I immediately fell into a state of empathy, which then drove my inquisitive mind to learn why she was in this hospital bed in this state. As details of her story were revealed to me over the coming months, in correlation with her elongated stay in hospital, I learnt the intricate narrative of her healthcare-seeking behaviour. It demonstrates clearly some of the challenges facing patients and doctors during healthcare decision-making processes.

Dechen was two years old when the farm road leading to Chali was cut into the mountainside by large bulldozers and a team of road workers. Standing in certain parts of Mongar, it was possible to follow the brown and grey scar of the road as it hugged the steep slope, framed by the dark green forest. It was rugged, but it was the only direct link to Chali. Although a better tarmac road that led to the northern Lhuntse *dzongkhag* ran below the village, it had not been connected due to topographic challenges. Thus the only other point of access was straight through the forested mountainsides that skirted the valley walls. The construction of this road would come to play an important role in Dechen's illness.

Dechen was enjoying life in her family home, where her parents worked their fields, eating what they grew and selling any remainder in the Mongar market. But soon after the road was built, something changed. Dechen's left arm began to ache, just below the elbow. An illness was not immediately obvious to her parents because the intensity and frequency of her pain was slow to set in. It caused her to cry sporadically, and she was growing increasingly irritable. Her parents tried feeding her more food, thinking she was hungry and tired, but it didn't seem to make a difference. Eventually her parents noticed she was continually motioning to the length of her left arm and complaining of pain and tenderness. She became protective over it, unwilling to let her parents touch it, and she eventually stopped using it to eat with and pick up toys, preferring her right arm to compensate. The parents then noticed the arm didn't look quite right, it had a strange bend or deformity. Although there was no wound or mark, it did occasionally flare up, becoming red, swollen and warm to touch, a clear indication that something inside the arm was wrong. After one month of these early signs of illness, she became anaemic, frail and pallid. She ran unexplained temperatures and had bouts of lethargy, nausea and fatigue.

Although they lived in a small intimate house and slept in the same room, as many farming families do in Bhutan, the slow onset of these symptoms played an important role in how Dechen's parents reacted. Young children stay very close to their mothers in the first few years of life. Many don't attend school until much later, and will be carried on their mothers' backs to fields, markets, kitchens, cattle pastures or wood-plenty forests. This proximity and gradual onset of symptoms meant that the parents didn't definitively realize anything was wrong. It was only with the build-up, repetition and patterning of symptoms after one month that they understood their daughter was not well.

Focus groups that I held with senior health assistants, most with ten to fifteen years' experience of working in rural BHUs, identified different first-response behaviours between patients with rapid onset symptoms and those whose symptoms came on slower. They identified two variables that generally affected a patient's or attendees's decision to visit a hospital.

The first variable is time. The quicker the onset, the more likely the first response will be a visit to a state healthcare institution. For example, sudden blindness would commonly cause patients to attend hospital immediately or within a few days given such complicating factors as transport, work duties or finances. However, patients who develop blindness over the course of weeks, months or years – as those with cataracts – may not arrive at hospital for months or years, if ever. I met one such blind man in Lingshi who could have benefitted greatly from the four-day trip to Thimphu Hospital, perhaps restoring his sight, but the family couldn't spare the labour, time or money to make such a trip. The Ministry of Health is aware of such issues, especially about blindness. As a result, hospital teams will occasionally travel to remote areas to perform cataract surgery in makeshift operating theatres. These teams commonly meet patients with chronic illnesses that chose not to respond by visiting a hospital or BHU.[3]

The second variable is severity of symptoms. Severe pain, visibly distressing ailments, bleeding, accidents, paralysis, convulsions and fits would force patients to a hospital within a few days – although broken bones, apparently severe enough, may not result in a hospital visit but rather one to a community bone-setter who would reset and splint the wound. This exception is especially common in more remote mountain regions where travel to BHUs is restricted by long distances or rugged landscape traversed by foot. In cases such as these, it may be more important to respond swiftly and decisively than to decide on which practice to use. But generally the more severe a symptom is considered to be, the more likely the patient or decision-maker will seek out hospital care.

Both these first-response drivers were acting against Dechen. Her symptoms were not severe at first, and they developed over a long time. Thus, her parents and those in her family home did not act quickly.

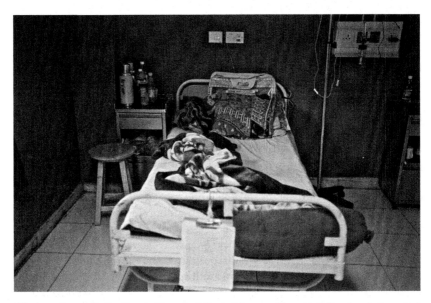

Illustration 3.7 Dechen's Hospital Bed, *Mongar Hospital*. Dechen's hospital bed awaits her return from surgery.

Clearly some aspects of Dechen's story are similar to those of Sonam and Tshomo's son's. First, the patients were both young and unable to make healthcare decisions for themselves. They were wards of their parents. While I researched decision-making processes with older patients who had greater command over their own care, I found that studying children and their parents offered a poignantly direct window into these processes. The level of suffering experienced by older patients was definitely a factor in when, where, how and why they would seek particular healthcare. Talking with adult patients who were suffering themselves, such as Pema from chapter 1, I learnt how pain was experienced and managed between differing practices, healths and bodies. However, pain and suffering could also obscure some of the other factors involved in a decision. Talking with parents about their young children as patients, I was able to learn about these other complicating factors in decisions without the shadow of pain experiences, even though both sets of parents were concerned and worried.

Second, as we will see, the practices being deliberated were again biomedical and religious. The practices could also be categorized as institutional and non-institutional, hospital and home, biomedical and alternative. While my ethnographic examples include deliberation over similar practices, there are many other practices for patients to decide among. For example, Pema used cutting and sucking; patients in chapter 2 chose the traditional medicine system; in chapter 4 we will learn about other more extreme alternative practices. Deliberation is not always between biomedical practices and an alternative – biomedical practice is not a constant. I met some patients who were deciding between different types of alternative healers, such as a shaman working on spirit possession or a finder of lost souls. Thus, while my two examples of child patients use similar religious and biomedical practices, the wider field of decision-making processes can involve any number and type of healing practices.

One major difference between my two cases marks how these parents ultimately made their healthcare-seeking decisions. As I will explain, Dechen's parents had a definite spiritual diagnosis in hand, whereas Sonam and Tshomo reeled in indecision. With a firm diagnosis, Dechen's parents were able to quickly identify a treatment for their daughter.

Dechen's father explained to me that in building the new road, a tree had been cut down. He said this tree had belonged to the village's *yül lha* (*yul lha*), translated roughly as 'village or territorial deity'. When its tree was cut down, the *yül lha* had been disturbed. Subsequently it sought reprisal. The father thought that it had chosen his daughter and specifically her arm as the target for this malevolent action. In some way, it was causing the breakdown of her body.

Such vengeful actions by malevolent spirits, ghosts, mountain deities, or other forms of spiritual beings are commonplace in Bhutan. Kunzang Choden (2008) gives an extensive briefing of the many variants of malevolent spirits in just one valley, Tang in Bumthang *dzongkhag*, demonstrating the complexity of spiritual categorizations and how each spirit requires a different propitiatory approach. Francoise Pommaret (2004) has written extensively on the territories and behaviours of such *yül lha*, emphasizing their linkages with kinship relations, areas of control, power and rituals. Riamsara Kuyakanon Knapp (2015) extends this work with a contemporary ethnography of mountain closure rituals and sacred geographies, exploring how the meaningful exchanges between mountain deities and local inhabitants are intimately related to environmental practices.

All of these works, as well as many others, highlight how human inhabitants of these territories are inextricably connected to deities and spirits and are constantly engaged in maintaining reciprocal and propitiatory relations. Pommaret (2004: 61–62) notes,

> It is quite impossible to give a definite pattern for the worship of the deity of the territory in Bhutan, but we can remark that albeit protean, it is alive and requires the participation of the whole community. . . . The deity of the territory emerges like an anthropomorphic lord ruling an estate with a large range of rights over individuals but also duties regarding their protection and well-being. If the deity also takes a function, as is often the case, of birth-deity, cattle-deity and warrior-deity, his or her powers over daily life are almost unlimited. In exchange, the people offer him or her rituals which are testimonies of allegiance, gifts, supplications and sublimated taxes, and they try not to break the social and physical order so that the lord is not offended.

Within this cosmological exchange between deities and persons, it's important to note that *yül lha* also plays a positive role in the ongoing life and work of a village. Sonam Kinga marks how amicable relations with a *yül lha* can bring positive effects in an ethnographic study he did in Yungtoed Valley in Lhuntse *dzongkhag* in the east (2008: 43):

> While Gortshom community alone propitiates the yue lha or village deities, the consequence of non-propitiation or provoking them can be harmful to all villages in Yungtoed valley. Similarly, the benefits of propitiation and appeasement can be enjoyed by all in the form of timely rainfall, absence of illness and misfortunes to both humans and livestock, and bumper harvests. The whole Yungtoed valley or villages under Metsho Gewog are under the protection of these yue lha, whom Gortshom community propitiates.

In Dechen's case, the 'physical order' of the landscape, and thus the *yül lha* that was that landscape, had been broken with the building of the new road. Given that she was of the village of Chali, following Pommaret's and Kinga's insights into the allegiances of persons and their mountain deities, clearly she was a territory of sorts, a human geography over which the *yül lha* had power, and thus she was a target of its vengeance.

It's noteworthy that Dechen had no agency in the building of the road or in her kinship relations. Although she was destined to benefit from its construction through easier access to Mongar, she herself had very little, if anything to do with its construction. However, this made no difference. As Pommaret (2004) notes, kinship relations are a fundamental connection between a person and their local deity. The parents believed that through these kinship lines, even though Dechen had not wielded the axe that cut the tree, the deity had punished her with illness. With this decision, it was clear to the parents and their community that they would have to hold indemnifying religious ceremonies to rectify the transgression.

At the start of the second month, the parents set to work on rituals to appease the *yül lha*. Setting up a religious ceremony, such as the *rim dro* that Sonam and Tshomo performed, is not as straightforward as it may seem – further decisions regarding the type of ritual await. The child's astrology, the particular deities involved, the religious institutions available, the time of year, the circumstances of the transgression and the severity of the case or symptoms are taken into account. Additionally, *rim dro* rituals are only one type of religious healing intervention, with many others complementing familial and community healthiness. To select a particular ritual, patients often visit a *lama* or astrologer who will collect information about the patient before deciding on a practice. This is a diagnosis of sorts, like consulting a biomedical general practitioner (GP) before seeing a specialist. Like many GPs, these religious diagnosticians will have their preferred religious practitioners carry out the ceremonies, so favourable social relations between practitioners is also a factor in deciding on a religious ritual. These individuals may also incorporate a biomedical or traditional element to their referral advice, sending patients to institutional services as well as alternative healers (see chapter 4).

Recalling Pommaret's (2004) statement that it is impossible to define a pattern of worship, the varying combinations of these factors make selection between types of ritual very challenging. From the patient perspective, deciding upon a religious or alternative practice is not a straightforward process. Instead there are multiple choices within a range of religious or spiritual healing practices. Most literature on patient behaviour in Bhutan from the Ministry of Health misses this point, preferring to see a binary between a single biomedical and single alternative treatment option (see introduction). But there are many choices along this alternative route, adding another layer of complication, a depth of choice that patients in Bhutan must learn to navigate and manage to find the appropriate cure. In trying to assemble an effective religious response to their child's illness, Dechen's parents enlisted their astrologer and *lama*, and all participated in selecting a type of *rim dro*.

The *rim dro* was enacted in the family home, with Dechen present. For several days the air was thick with incense, cymbals and drums were beaten, cyclical mantra were recited throughout all hours, offerings were given, food was prepared for both the deity and the *lamas*, funds were given to the practitioners for their efforts, and the parents hoped for the best.

A week passed, but sadly Dechen's symptoms continued.

The father recounted to me his dismay that the ritual hadn't worked and that his daughter's condition had worsened. He told me that after discussing the matter with his wife and village *lama*, they concluded that the ritual had been wrong and another type would be tried. Again the *rim dro*, but again it took no effect. A third was conducted, and again no change. Three months passed and Dechen's illness hadn't abated. By now the temperatures, lethargy, nausea and fatigue confined her to bed. With little success from the religious treatment route, they decided to try the hospital across the valley.

This was a crucial change in the decision-making process and, according to my focus groups with health assistants as well as many interviews with doctors and nurses, one that many other patients repeat every day in Bhutan. A change in treatment routes is common, especially after the trial and failure of another practice. For example, Pema from chapter 1 changed to the institutional form of traditional medicine after her nasal pain resurfaced and, in her view, biomedicine failed to address the problem. Given the multiple practices available to Bhutanese patients, such trial and error is a productive part of healthcare-seeking behaviour.

At these decision-making junctures it's tempting to think that Dechen's parents made a cognitive switch and dismissed as wrong their original notions of causation regarding the deity or that they now believed religious intervention to be inadequate or inappropriate as a cure. However, the parents in this case did not make such drastic changes in opinion. Rather than rejecting the religiosity of the illness and replacing it with a biomedical interpretation, the religious understanding still thrived, this time entangled with a biomedical practice. This also meant that the decision-making process was not between this practice or that practice, but how to organize and assemble a healing response that best approached the various dimensions of the patient multiple. This recalls my argument from chapter 1 that explored how Bhutanese patients live in multiple and simultaneous subjectivities of 'patient-hood' in relation to the practices they engage with. To understand this more fully and how such melding of ideologies makes decision-making a complex and multilayered process, let me first explain what happened at Mongar Hospital.

When the orthopaedic surgeon examined Dechen, he quickly identified the illness as osteomyelitis, a well-known and researched biomedical disease type in which bone marrow develops an infection and inflammation. *Robbins Basic Pathology* (Kumar et al. 2012: 773–74) gives the following explanation:

> Most cases of acute osteomyelitis are caused by bacteria. The offending organisms reach the bone by one of three routs: (1) hematogenous dissemination (most common); (2) extension from an infection in adjacent joint or soft tissue; or (3) traumatic implantation after compound fractures or orthopaedic procedures. . . . Osteomyelitis classically manifests as an acute systemic illness, with malaise, fever, leukocytosis, and throbbing pain over the affected region. Symptoms can also be subtle with only unexplained fever, particularly in infants, or only localized pain in the adult.

With four months of the infection festering in her arm, Dechen had reached a critical state of malaise. She was prepped for surgery and two days later was under anaesthesia having her bone cracked open and the infected marrow drained. As successful as this surgery was, the biomedical doctor explained to the parents that their daughter would now require a long and strong course of antibiotics to fight the return of the infection. Dechen lay in her hospital bed in the large open ward for the next month while her parents stayed with her. Eventually she recovered from the surgery and showed good signs of improvement, and she was permitted to return home.

The visiting orthopaedic surgeon from North America who was treating Dechen with his Bhutanese resident counterpart explained to me that osteomyelitis is often a chronic disease that can be very challenging to cure outright. Most patients require continued and lengthy treatment, sometimes over the course of years, during which flare-ups and resurgences of infection and symptoms are common. Dechen followed this chronic path and was back in hospital only a month later with the same symptoms. Again she underwent surgery and a course of antibiotics, staying in hospital for another month. Again she returned home, fell ill and was brought back to hospital. This is where I found her, about to enter her third surgery, one that was going to be more invasive than the last two, which would leave her arm deformed for life.

Let's now return to the issues of decision-making between biomedical and religious routes, specifically how choosing to visit a hospital doesn't render insignificant the religiosity of the illness, as perceived by patients and their carers. Repeated treatments for the resurgence of symptoms were traumatic for Dechen and her parents. The month-long hospital stays strained the family and threw their farm labour into disarray. It also put a financial burden on the household; although the hospital treatments were free, there was still the cost of the *rim dro*, the loss of farm income, the purchase of food while in Mongar and the cost of transport. But regardless of these costs, the family continued to bring Dechen back to hospital when symptoms worsened. Having tried a religious-only route, they were now dependent on biomedical healthcare. However, during the months at home or in hospital, they continued to perform *rim dro* and other religious rituals that engaged in reciprocity with the *yül lha*. This form of alternative care continued simultaneously throughout months spent in the hospital. How did the parents conceive of Dechen's illness in the context of her biomedical care and disease interpretation? What might this reveal about decision-making processes and the idea of 'appropriate care'?

I explicitly asked the father why he thought his daughter's illness was abating in hospital and returning at home. He explained in a matter-of-fact way that the transgression of the deity's home and subsequent dishonouring was still causing his daughter's disease. Yes, osteomyelitis was what the doctors called it, and yes, he understood, in a limited way, the scientific explanation and subsequent treatment methodology, but this was a secondary rationale. The original cause was the malevolence of their village deity. The symptoms, as described by the doctors, were just that: 'symptoms' of the deity's actions interpreted by doctors. Furthermore, he hypothesized that in taking his daughter to hospital and travelling the distance away from their village, mountainside and the deity's territory, the deity's power was diminished. In this disempowered state, the doctors' medicine, which he genuinely thought of as highly effective, could abate the symptoms. But on returning to the territory, the power of the deity was at its peak and it could easily reimpose the illness. This logic that placed the cause of the illness in the relationship between *yül lha* and family demanded that propitiation continue whether Dechen was being treated in hospital or not.

The father's rationale regarding the power of deities within and beyond their 'territories' is a transmutable notion, open for interpretation, variance and disparity within the Mongar and Bhutan contexts. On discovering this story, I originally became excessively excited about how this logic might apply in public health programming. Doctors have long complained about the delay in first-response healthcare-seeking behaviours. In Dechen's example, the doctors were adamant that if the parents had brought her in at the first onset of symptoms, they might have saved her great suffering and a disfigurement. The delay of three months was catastrophic for the disease's progression and severity. Efforts to dissuade people from religious or alternative treatments are obviously not very effective, for even if biomedicine offered a cure, a patient's view of causality remained with the religious interpretation. As one surgeon put it, 'I completed a massive five-hour operation on a patient, and when I told their family that it had been successful and the patient would survive, they ran off to thank their *lama* for saving him!' Perhaps then a public service announcement could promote both a religious- and biomedical-first response. It might read: 'In Pain? Come to hospital immediately and perform *rim dro* at home. After all, the further away you are from that malevolent deity, the less power he has over you!' I fantasized about solving a mega public health issue in Bhutan, applying my research in such a strategic way as to support both religious beliefs and institutionalized healthcare.

However my enthusiasm was short-lived. One quick, counter-ethnographic story a month later brought me up short: A Bhutanese man had travelled to Geneva, Switzerland, on business and fallen ill, landing him in hospital. His family and community back in Thimphu described how he had rudely forsaken his village *yül lha*, failing to make the appropriate offerings before his travel, thinking himself above and beyond such allegiances, especially while abroad in Europe. Unfortunately for him, this was not the case, and the deity followed him and made him ill. It appears that the powers of deities are not limited to their territories; they operate through a human geography as well, following their subjects through valleys, *dzongkhags* and across international borders.

Both Kuyakanon (2015) and Pommaret (2004) explore the issues of territorial space, with the latter touching on the idea of deity migration (2004: 50–51) and control of space and residence. In the face of this contradicting ethnographic story and with the work of Pommaret and Kuyakanon, as well as many others in the Tibetan (Samuel 1993: 184), Bhutan (Bodt 2012) and Nepal (Lim 2008: 174–75) regions, it appears the activities and behaviours of deities such as *yül lha* are far too complex and transient for such a narrow public health announcement as the one I had envisioned. Although my enthusiasm fell flat, the evidence and analytical work only proves further that patients in Bhutan are entangled in multiple health, practice and aetiological narratives that will often run simultaneous to each other, yet all require meaningful and time-consuming engagement. Hence the decision-making processes of patients between practices are equally complex, and often times mutually informed. In this example, Dechen's parents saw the biomedical explanation for the illness as part of the illness's religious aspects. The two were mutually inclusive.

Conclusion: The Conundrum of Appropriate Care

Having fleshed out two ethnographic narratives of healthcare-seeking behaviour and the complex decision-making processes that defined them, I want to turn my attention to the very challenging and much-debated issue of 'appropriate care' within the Bhutanese context.

Clearly the healthcare-seeking behaviour of most Bhutanese is changing rapidly. New health services, communication channels, media exposure and transport are but a few of the factors influencing patients to seek healthcare in new ways. While little is known about healthcare and patient decision-making

before the 1960s and the introduction of the biomedical and traditional institutionalized practices, we do know that patients would have had to settle with
only healers and community remedies. The arrival of institutionalized medicine
and pharmaceuticals has significantly complicated the decision-making process
for patients where the range of healing choices has expanded and a new ethics
of 'appropriate behaviour' when it comes to seeking care has emerged. We have
seen two detailed examples in this chapter where decision-makers have debated
various practice responses to illness. We have also explored some of the factors
that influence the decisions they make, such as finances, topography, diagnosis
recognition, illness onset characteristics and symptom severity. These factors
along with the practices themselves shape ethical discourse over when, where,
how and why to seek a particular treatment.

One of the loudest voices in this ethical discourse is the Ministry of Health,
its doctors and its proponents. The institutional arm of this voice is the public
health programming department of the ministry, yet this is just one formalized
voice. The more powerful, pervasive and abundant voice is that of the doctors,
nurses and staff themselves. Their agenda is to get patients to turn to the biomedical or traditional services in all instances of illness. Tshomo's pregnancy,
for example, in the opinion of the gynaecological doctor in Mongar Hospital, is
a matter for the hospital and the hospital only. According to the orthopaedic
doctor, Dechen may have avoided disfigurement had the biomedical services
been consulted first. I do not wish to argue the validity of such claims here but
to emphasize the types of practice-centric ethics being spread by these interlocutors. Backing them up are newspapers, television programming, public
health education, and more often than not, the younger generations that have
grown up within state schooling systems that promote hospital attendance.
Undoubtedly it was some form of this agenda that inspired Dechen's parents to
eventually take their daughter to hospital rather than try the fourth *rim dro*.

The alternative voice of care is non-coalesced, non-institutional and thus
de-centralized. It's the voice of all the alternative healers and the patients that
believe in their remedies; it's the local mountain deities that cause and ameliorate illness; it's the Buddhist histories that inform the inner contours of suffering, the tastes of home-prepared remedies and oral traditions of familial care;
it's the agentive meaningfulness given to one's own interpretation of why one is
ill, regardless of which science, tradition, history, proof or academic institution
it sits in. The easiest people to point to here are the alternative healers and
religious practitioners that have been explored in this ethnography, but it
ranges further than that. The de-centring conceptions of health, practice and
body that make up the patients of Bhutan have their own place and meaningfulness in the healing narratives, and they exert a power too. This is what drove
Tshomo and Sonam to stall in making a decision for their son; it's what made
Dechen endure months of screaming, fever and suffering. These powers of
alternative-healing discourse are real in that people live by the ethics and
knowledge they propound.

These agendas and their proponents are not always maligned. As we saw with Sonam and Tshomo, people are finding new ways to allow seemingly contrasting discourses to simultaneously assert their power in everyday healing narratives, altering behaviours and practices but in a complementary fashion. This was highlighted by an alternative healer I worked with in Mongar who said that after performing some very invasive healing rituals, further discussed in chapter 4, he would tell patients to immediately visit the hospital. 'Why not?' he asked. 'It couldn't hurt.' Therefore while ethical positions of appropriate behaviour are being fought over, there is a dynamic of compatibility that offers hope for the future of medical pluralism in Bhutan.

However, in the wake of arguments surrounding 'appropriate care' and 'appropriate healthcare-seeking behaviour', I think there is a serious threat to the current position of medical pluralism in Bhutan. With global medical assemblages reaching more powerful network nodes within health institutions and government (see Ong and Collier 2004a, b; Ong 2005), biomedicine and its ethics of care are increasingly taking ground away from smaller, more alternative proponents. New legislation in Bhutan's constitution is taking hold, requiring state-run hospitals and ministries to take more control over the types of practices available in Bhutan. The ministry has made fledgling efforts to require all alternative healers to register under the Bhutan Medical and Health Council, the agency responsible for legalizing, certifying and monitoring doctors, surgeons, nurses, and others. Although these efforts are cursory, with little ability to implement such policy, the trajectory is clear. Anything 'health' related should be controlled, monitored and authorized by the central government. There are even discussions at the ministry level about how to incorporate religious healers and healing rituals into such certification policy. The traditional medicine services could play a key role in this, as noted in recent comments by the National Traditional Medicine Hospital superintendent in a *Kuensel* article: 'We're planning to train them [alternative healers] about the importance of health and hygiene while practicing. . . . We're planning to preserve such practices and issue certificates to the good ones' (*Kuensel* 2013). At the patient and practitioner level the call for certification and authorization is starting to take effect too. One alternative healer refused to talk to me, stating that he was already embroiled in multiple civil lawsuits with past patients and he didn't want to risk entangling himself further in these growing punitive powers (see chapter 4 for more details).

Developments in healthcare centralization and control arise from various motivational factors. As the patient demand for better biomedical and traditional state services increases, so too do things like physician malpractice cases, rigorous morbidity reporting, programme evaluations, performance metrics, health and safety standards, national health policies (MoH 2011b), civil rights legislation, transparency monitoring and accountability checks. All of these mobilizing pressures are driving health institutions to strengthen their arguments, efforts and tactics towards biomedical and traditional dominance. A good example is the Drug Regulatory Authority, whose director explained to me that the reason his agency is so stringent in monitoring alternative healers' medications and prescriptions is that it is their legal mandate to do so (DRA 2012 and 2013a). Such institutions take their emerging democracy and elected powers very seriously and aim to fulfil the legislation set up to guide them, regardless of any resulting teething problems; the massive drug shortages discussed in chapter 5 are a good example. Such motives drive the agenda of the Ministry of Health and its international partners (non-governmental organizations and government financial sponsors) to centralize and standardize healthcare in Bhutan under the auspices of its institutionalized forms of care, thus asserting a particular ethic of what is appropriate care and healthcare-seeking behaviour.

The obvious risk to alternative healers is drowning in this ethical discourse. *Lamas, rim dro,* shamanic healers, religious practitioners, spirit possessors, mediums, oracles, cutters and suckers, burners with hot iron, deities, *yül lha,* retired *drungtsho,* community practitioners, family dieticians and bone-setters: what space will they have to continue their offerings? What might happen to the healths, practices and bodies they create and heal? How will the ethics that at present support these practices fade away in the face of a more dominant response to illness?

Mol's (2008) work in *The Logic of Care: Health and the Problem of Patient Choice* might find productive space for the institutional and non-institutional to collaborate in treating patients effectively. She argues that 'introducing patient choice into healthcare does not . . . make space for us, its patients. Instead, it alters daily practices in ways that do not necessarily fit well with the intricacies of our diseases' (2008: 18). In her ethnographic context of diabetes care in and around a 'university hospital in a medium-sized Dutch town' (33), as well as other fieldsites, she argues against healthcare approaches that promote 'choice' for patients rather than 'care'. She calls the systemic approach of encouraging multiples of treatment options a 'logic of choice' that ultimately fails to address the variable needs of patients. Instead she argues 'that the tradition of care contains more suitable repertoires for handling life with a disease. Instead of frustrating these by dreaming of choice, it would be wiser to try to improve care on its own terms. In its own terms' (18). For Mol, a 'logic of care' aims to provide services that match patient needs rather than their freedoms of choice.

Her argument is persuasive in that within a logic of care patients would theoretically receive the most effective treatment to match their illness. Her argument works well in contexts where a single form of medicine prevails, such as biomedicine in its treatment of diabetes or HIV (see for example McKechnie 1999 or Okely 1999). Within this unidimensional healthcare setting, services could refocus on care rather than choice, realigning principles and delivery of services such as pharmaceuticals (Mol 2008: 215) that Petryna et al. (2006) have convincingly shown to take advantage of wide parameters of choice, specifically within global pharmaceutical markets. Perhaps logics of care would rid markets of pharmaceutical over-saturation and provide targeted and more efficient channels to healing.

But what happens in a practice-plural context like Bhutan, where institutional and non-institutional healing agents diversify choice but often don't work together? I argue that a reworking of Mol's logics of care and choice might offer a way to see medical pluralism as a viable and ultimately effective way forwards. She theorizes (2008: 176),

> For no matter how loudly the wonders of patient choice are celebrated, I am not so optimistic. My worry is that, with the introduction of patient choice, many other things get fixed as well: the circumstances in which we make our choices; the alternatives between which we may choose; the boundaries around the 'care products' we may or may not opt for; and so on. Fixing all of these things would frustrate doctoring, as it would make it even more difficult to attune the various viscous variables relevant in care to each other. What is more, 'choice' comes with many hierarchical dichotomies that are foreign to 'care': active versus passive; health versus disease; thinking versus action; will versus fate; mind versus body. Bringing these dichotomies into play is not going to improve the lives of people with a disease, if only because they end up time and again on the wrong side of the divide.

She gets to the heart of the tension in both Sonam and Tshomo's and Dechen's narratives; in contexts of multiple practice, patients' decisions become 'fixed' and delineated between their choices. The rhetoric of the biomedical institution against alternative practices is one of many 'fixing' agents, pinpointing an 'other' and asserting its disagreement with its otherness. This fixing and delineation creates the contrasting ethics of 'appropriate care' that cause dangerous situations of choice, such as the ones Sonam and Tshomo faced. In situations of this or that, biomedical or alternative, biomedical or traditional, traditional or alternative, bone-setter or spirit possessor, nutriceutical or pharmaceutical, milk or honey, it's the oscillation between two practices and the invariable isolation of one that brings risks to patients. Mol insists that these choices are not only confusing for patients to navigate but also, in and of themselves, reduce the chances of patients receiving effective treatments. This is a statement that almost all practitioners – alternative, biomedical or traditional – would agree with.

How then might Bhutan learn from Mol's idea of logics of care without totally disbanding its medical pluralism, its practice, health and body multiples that make up the patient multiple, the diversity that essentially gives life and meaning to so many people, in illness and in daily life?

I would argue that medical pluralism is essential to the identity of many Bhutanese. If not always essential for effective treatment, it does allow people to express their identities, their culture, their experiences of suffering and healing, and their phenomenologies of pain. Pema from chapter 1 demonstrated just that. The practice, health and body multiples that thrive in Bhutan provide meaning to patients and their communities. The variants of these multiples are the markers of a healing sociality, but they also denote a wider cultural awareness. Therefore, the preservation of this diversity helps people express who they are, breathes life into their daily lives, most acutely through their experiences of suffering and amelioration. If the goal is to preserve this meaningfulness and heal people, then the application of a logic of care requires the preservation of a plural practice context without the need to delineate and divide practices between an ethic. In other words, the logic of care in Bhutan would require a diverse set of practices that can approach the many different needs of Bhutanese patients.

This is a tall order. How can we avoid the production of practice-centric ethics, such that are argued by doctors, media, alternative healers and traditional *drungtsho*? I see a solution to this question and the hopeful future of Bhutan's medical context in the simultaneous enactment of all practices, supported by a logic of care. Sonam and Tshomo demonstrated this future when they conducted *rim dro* and went to hospital. They demonstrated the capacity to not decide between one practice or another but to select both. Dechen's parents made slightly different decisions, taking longer to visit hospital, resulting in severe complications. It wasn't so much a case of one practice or another but rather whether or not to visit hospital. In a logic of care it is this latter deliberation that should be targeted. Getting patients to come to hospital quickly is not rejecting other practices but rather insisting for a better logic of care in the decision-making processes of patients. Therefore I argue that healthcare services should be less concerned with discriminating against other practices and focus on persuasion tactics through a logic of effective care. Undoubtedly it will be the coming generations who will decide whether they will adopt multiple practices and use them alongside each other. We know of other cultures, communities and nations that have done something similar; Arthur Kleinman (1981), Leslie (1976) and Leslie and Young (1992) are good historical examples, with Kim (2003) and Craig et al. (2010) offering more contemporary reflections.

An issue highlighted by many of these authors in the practical application of medical pluralism concerns the contradictions that arise between alternative and biomedical practices. My study of the ethics of appropriate care demonstrates how these contradictions are discussed by doctors and patients. It also shows the dangerous potential of treatment delay, as in the case of Sonam and Tshomo. However, Kim, in his work *Korean Shamanism: The Cultural Paradox* (2003: 18), highlights a potential way to sidestep these frictions and ethical discordance:

> I have discovered throughout this study that I was wrong in 1988. The characteristics of Korean shamanism are so intrinsically different from those of medical modalities that it would cause great confusion not only for health practitioners, but also for ordinary Koreans, if Shamanism was included in health planning as a health-care resource. Nor do shamans work in the field of health care (or the health-care sector) where medical practitioners work. Medical treatment and the shaman's ritual business are quite different from each other . . . I never heard shamans complain that they should be treated as traditional medical practitioners, nor that they should be given medical licences.

This finding resounds almost verbatim in my own ethnographic findings. Although the category of 'shamans' does not translate smoothly between Kim's ethnographic context and my own, the distinct social and professional spaces for institutional healthcare providers and alternative healers were marked in the attitudes of patients, healers and doctors. Many alternative healers were not considered to be healthcare practitioners, although they definitely were sought after when illness occurred. To collapse these two would, as Kim notes, be erroneous and possibly confusing for healthcare practitioners and patients. It was the patients and their illnesses that travelled between practices, not the practices themselves.

It is this very gap that might offer the solution of a viable medical pluralism in Bhutan. If the modalities of practice can remain distinct rather than in contrast and contention, patients and health policy might find a way to effectually use this diversity. This would fundamentally change the decision-making processes of patients. Dechen's parents would not decide between choices, but decide to use all of them. Ridding the 'either/or' component safeguards the Ministry of Health's agenda to get more patients to come to hospital promptly and encourage the cultural, personal and healing agency of other practices. Arguments over which practice is better to cure which disease – i.e. the ethics of appropriate care – become practically redundant in this scenario, for each is caring for the patient in its own way. By pursuing a logic of care, Bhutan might be able to claim to propagate a multi-practice healing scenario in which patients may thrive.

Notes

1. The use of stirrup support in deliveries has increased over the past decade as stirrup equipment has made its way into BHUs around the country. Use of such medical equipment during childbirth has had much attention in medical anthropology. For example Emily Martin (2001) describes the ways in which women's bodies are conceived by biomedical practices. She looks at biomedicine's mechanization of women's bodies and the subsequent use of birthing tools like stirrups and forceps in the delivery process. Her critical analysis of biomedicine's conception of women's bodies questions these methods of delivery, offering examples of other less painful or intrusive methods. Unfortunately for many mothers in Bhutan, the mechanization of women's bodies so often attributed to biomedical methods is very much under development in BHUs as a part of standardizing delivery nationwide. This wasn't always the case. Traditional medicine *thangkas* describing childbirth (Cai et al. 2008) show methods of delivery such as squatting and on hands and knees. Such practices have evidently been used for a long time and offer an alternative to the methods used in BHUs. More research into birthing methods is sorely needed to help the Ministry of Health devise forward-thinking birthing strategies that find the best solutions for Bhutanese mothers.
2. Although I use the term 'village' here, the spacing, formation and layout of such community settlements can be vastly different from the typical villages known in the UK or North. As Pommaret (2004: 40) notes,

A 'village' was traditionally composed of several clusters of houses, sometimes a distance of one hour's walk from each other. It was, in fact, an area coming under one general name, and each cluster of houses had its own name. A yul [village] is therefore quite similar to the now outdated connotation of the French word 'pays', meaning not the country but the region of origin, and found in the old colloquial expression 'on est pays', 'we are from the same region/village'. In the Bhutanese conception of living space, one could therefore say that the reference unit is the *yul.*

3. This is also confirmed in an interview conducted in Thimphu with a leading Bhutanese ophthalmologist, who frequented these trips.

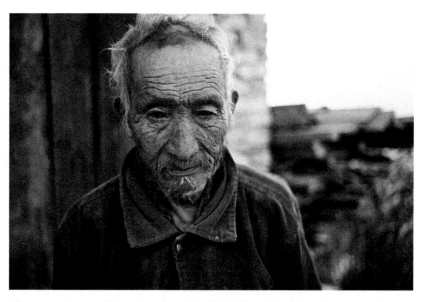

Illustration 4.1 A Returner of Lost Souls, *Mongar.* Yeshi, an alternative healer, specializes in the returning of lost souls. He is not a *ja né* healer.

4

Alternative Practices and the Removal of *Ja Né*

Introducing Alternative Practices

The aim of this chapter is to explore how patients in Bhutan are affected by some of the alternative practices they use. As described in chapter 1, 'alternative practices' include, but are not limited to, activities such as shamanism, bone-setting, cutting and sucking, poison removal, spirit possession, dietary changes and other non-institutionalized healing practices. This chapter begins looking into these practices through a wide angle of view and then narrows to a specific disease known as *ja né* (orthographic forms follow later in the chapter) and how it is healed. To understand how alternative practices affect patients, we must also explore some of the political and social pressures that in turn define the practice, knowledge and roles of these healers in their communities. Therefore, this chapter looks at the effect of practice on both healers and patients.

The first section discusses how some alternative healers operate within and around Mongar. It describes some of the variance found between practitioners and how this practice variance is utilized by patients. Emerging from the relationships between healer and patient are some of the wider political and social themes that play out in discourses of alternative healers in Bhutan. Specifically the section covers how healers are not isolated healthcare providers but rather part of a wider care network made up of intricate social relations and health knowledge.

An important caveat regarding the applicability of the findings of this chapter must be included here. The diversity of alternative healers in Bhutan is vast. Not only are there stark differences in alternative practices between urban and rural populations but also from east to west, valley to valley, village to village, household to household. It would be impossible and naive to think this chapter could accurately and sufficiently detail and apply all findings to this incredible diversity of practice and belief. Only recently in the last five years have anthropologists and other disciplines begun to explore the world of Bhutan's alternative healers, literature that is discussed below. The first section of this chapter thus offers a very brief and cursory overview of alternative healers and only some of the political contexts in which they operate.

The second section begins an ethnographic exploration into *ja né*, a disease 'category' that surfaced countless times during my fieldwork, with patients interpreting and responding to its symptoms, sufferings, healing and dying. There appears to be no published work to date on *ja né*, which is surprising given its frequency in my experiences across Bhutan. I open this ethnographic subject for further research in detailing three different uses of the term that I identified, all of which affect the ways that patients and the general populace think about illness and health. Again, it must be stressed that instances of *ja né* can be varied across Bhutan, and the ethnography presented here is limited to my fieldsites of Mongar, Thimphu and surrounding rural regions. Furthermore, *ja né* is only one of many disease types occurring within the alternative practice sphere and one that highlights the complexity and contentiousness of some alternative practices. There remain many other diseases, practices and healer types that could be further explored in Bhutan.

The final section details how one of these types of *ja né* was healed by an alternative healer. The practitioner, in Mongar, removed *ja né* from both male and female patients by using a sucking method from the genitalia. The practice had a level of vulnerability, exposure and tentative explicitness unlike anything else I observed in Bhutan. Subsequently, this practice that was well-known by many of my informants across Bhutan had garnered much popular interest, some of it sceptical. I explore this through a few examples of contentious incidents.

The chapter concludes by looking at the differing opinions surrounding the 'appropriateness' of *ja né* healing in relation to the ethnography presented. I argue that it's important to explore the ethnographic description of *ja né* practices and the contextualizing ethical discourses. I do so without applying my own ethical judgements to these practices. Such a neutral stance enables the first task of recording in academic scholarship the existence of this disease type within this very specific occurrence within my fieldwork data. It also helps this disease to exist in its own terms. Conclusive ethical judgements attached at this early stage may undermine the realities in which *ja né* plays out for patients and healers.

Medical anthropology and the discipline at large, as well as many other academic, medical and area-specific studies, have taken interest in non-biomedical alternative practices, producing a vast library of resources that spans histories (Saillant and Genest 2006), worldwide fieldsites (Singer and Erickson 2011), theories (Good et al. 2010) and application (Singer and Baer 2011), to name a few. Such works demonstrate the diversity and breadth of alternative healing practices and focus on the meaningful, agentive and complex roles they play in experiences of health, illness and healing.

While a literature review of the wider field of medical anthropology relating to alternative practices could only be sweeping and cursory, the lacuna of research and resources in the Bhutanese context make it possible to summarize the work completed thus far. Most of the literature written on alternative healers has focused on rituals and cultural practices, published by predominantly Bhutanese authors. Although the focus is not always on healing or healthcare, this work has added valuable insight into certain case studies of rituals that involve healers. Pommaret (2009), in her summative chapter '"Local Community Rituals" in Bhutan: Documentation and Tentative Reading' notes that the first of these Bhutanese-authored papers on rituals were from the 1980s (Wangmo 1985 and R. Dorji 1987), followed shortly by a series of papers in the early twenty-first century (D. T. Dorji [1999] 2008, 2002; Choden [1999] 2008; Pelgen 2000). The Centre for Bhutan Studies in Thimphu made a major contribution to the study of Bhutanese rituals with their 2004 publication *Wayo, Wayo* (CBS 2004), which collated works delineating the differences between local rituals (Pommaret 2009: 113). Continued publications in newspapers such as the *Bhutan Observer* and *Kuensel*, as well as an intangible cultural heritage project by the Institute of Language and Culture Studies (ILCS et al. 2006) funded by UNESCO, constitute a thriving knowledge base on ritual practices across Bhutan.

These works approach alternative healing practices tangentially to their focus on wider socio-cultural themes; only a few works look specifically at healing practices and practitioners. Of these, Tandin Dorji has written two of the best-known ethnographic works. His chapter 'The Spider, the Piglet and the Vital Principle: A Popular Ritual for Restoring the Srog' (2004) tells of a practice I too encountered where leaves are shaken over the head of the patient, upon which a white spider may fall, signifying the returning of a lost soul. Another of his articles, 'Acquiring Power: A Modality of Becoming a Pawo (dpa 'bo)' (2007), details the cosmological and practical aspects of *pawo* and *pamo* healers who are possessed by local deities to diagnose and treat patients. The latter will feature in this chapter.

More recently, Mona Schrempf has conducted extensive ethnographic research in the east of Bhutan and published several chapters that explore 'the complex landscape of ritual healers found in eastern Bhutan (Trashigang and Trashiyangtse Dzongkhags)' (Schrempf 2015a). Her chapter 'Spider, Soul, and Healing in Eastern Bhutan' (Schrempf 2015a) goes into further ethnographic detail than Dorji on the 'soul retrieval rite in which spiders serve as a ritual go-betweens, bridging human and other realms of local spirits and gods' (1). She has also written about the possession of spirit-mediums by Gesar, a powerful warrior king and mythical figure in both Bhutan and Tibetan traditions (Schrempf 2015b, c), again in eastern Bhutan. Her research gives valuable unexplored detail to the richness and specificity of alternative healers. Again, her work serves to demonstrate how localized and specific alternative healers in Bhutan can be and, thus, how researchers must be careful in applying findings too broadly. Through more research we can only begin to understand the complexity and interconnectedness of these alternative practices.

It is at this juncture – understanding the complex relations between alternative healers and their patients within a wider context of Bhutan's medical context – that this chapter aims to add to the literature. It explores where healers intersect both patients and wider socialities, politics and economies of health and healthcare, especially the institutionalized forms of biomedical and traditional medicine. While other authors have offered valuable case studies of particular practices and the cosmologies in which they operate, there is still much work to be done to locate these practices in the wider social or cultural networks of care that almost all patients use, sometimes simultaneously. This chapter sets out to follow such good examples of ethnographic detailing as the work of Schrempf (2015a–c) and T. Dorji (2004, 2007). In addition, it will add insight into the effect of alternative healing practices on patients and to contextualize these practices more broadly.

Power, Pressure and Demand

As I approached the end of my stay in Mongar I had accumulated information from interviews, conversations and observation sessions with alternative healers from the town and its surrounding communities. I was working with Singye, a traditional medicine *drungtsho* from the Mongar Hospital, who had proved an invaluable research partner. Singye had extensive knowledge and experience of healthcare, both inside and outside the *sowa rigpa* and biomedical practices. He had been a practitioner of *sowa rigpa* and a patient of both medicines for long periods of time. Additionally, he was very effective in arranging meetings with non-institutionalized practitioners. He was open, sympathetic and accepting of other ways of curing illness, and he encouraged the patients who used them, unlike some other traditional and biomedical doctors I knew. We worked well together, often eating at each other's houses, although his family environment and food was always more of a pleasure than my austere hospital bachelor quarters and survival diet. Through the course of our partnership, he had become a good ethnographer, understanding the questions we were looking to answer, and how to ask them to spur our informants to talk at length about their experiences, vulnerabilities, pain, families, opinions, gossip and any other interesting goings on from their healing narratives. For all these reasons I was feeling particularly confident when Singye and I strolled into a small roadside village thirty minutes outside of Mongar in search of Tandin, an alternative healer I had heard much about.

It was rumoured that Tandin could predict exam results, perhaps even the questions. He also offered an assortment of curative practices. His particular specialty was dealing with *ngan (ngen)*, poisonings or ill luck wished upon families at the behest of a rival, usually from a neighbouring village or community. As a result, Tandin dealt with some social causations of illness; bad relationships and long-standing feuds could instigate life-threatening diseases. He was

a social nexus of sorts; he resolved tensions and ills wrought by everyday contentious social relations. Needless to say, I was truly anticipating a meeting with
him.

It didn't go according to plan. By the end of our encounter with Tandin,
Singye and I were hightailing it off his land under threat of attack and condem-
nation. We hadn't even made it through the doorway. We were forbidden to
enter, declared antagonists, rejected as uninvited guests and offered no hospitality. I had heard of a harsher side to the Bhutanese, but I only witnessed it this
one time during my entire year in Bhutan. We had crossed a line of reasonable-
ness for Tandin, who sat in his darkened kitchen, swatting us away with aggres-
sive language and belligerent disgruntlement. I hadn't even been able to hand
over the customary bag of fluorescent juices, Druk Beer and sugary biscuits that
I brought to every interview as a gift. His animosity was clear and direct. As
much as this angered Singye, who expected a more gracious welcome, we both
decided to give up and leave quickly before threats of violence became actual.

Why did this happen and what can it tell us about the state of alternative
practices and their practitioners in Bhutan? First, I must confess to some irre-
sponsible decisions on my part that amateurishly positioned both Singye and
me negatively for Tandin. I had pushed Singye to take me to him without a
direct connection, invitation or introduction. Although Singye agreed – we had
had success with such approaches in the past – in hindsight I think even he
found this approach too forward. Slight acquaintances, indirect introductions,
shared friends, coincidences, karmic destinies, all these were things that might
have made us 'knowable' to this healer. We had none. To put it bluntly, we were
rude. It was a Bhutanese house visit equivalent to cold calling, and we were
hung up on quickly. But the healer's attitude sprang from more than our
discourtesy.

Even though Singye was a traditional *drungtsho* and was therefore hypo-
thetically more sensitive to alternative practices than a biomedical doctor, he
still worked at the hospital, the symbolic institution of centralized government
medicine. When he identified himself as a worker from hospital, a wall went up.
We became a threat. Singye tried to convey our interest, empathy and history
with other alternative healers in the area, as well as his own practice of *sowa
rigpa*, but he failed to dissuade the healer of our hostility. Tandin said earlier
approaches like ours had ended badly for him. He claimed he no longer
employed any type of alternative practices, even though I had met some of his
patients only recently in the hospital.

Afterwards I inquired around Mongar and the hospital into Tandin's recent
history. I learnt about his embroilment in a civil lawsuit. A family from a nearby
village was suing him on the grounds of slander. Apparently he had cured a
patient's illness by identifying a malevolent neighbour who had administered
ngan by a black magic called *tu* (*mthu*). Such dangers are ever-present for those
in the Mongar region; people use protective objects and religious rituals to
pre-empt such magic. Word soon spread about this malicious neighbour and

the *ngan* they 'blew' towards the patient. The neighbour vehemently disagreed with the accusations, and sued Tandin for defamation, claiming the entire family's reputation had been damaged. Furthermore, the lawsuit had gained the attention of the Ministry of Health, and the healer had been targeted as an 'unauthorized' and 'unaccredited' healthcare practitioner. He was at further risk of fines and the loss of income from not being able to practice freely.

It was no wonder then that Tandin considered Singye and me a risk. Singye's affiliation with the hospital, my 'researcher' status and the general rudeness of our uninvited visit were enough to put him on the defensive. For many other alternative healers that I spoke to, their current default political position was defensive. While they were open, willing and proud to talk about their healing craft, almost all identified how difficult it was becoming to practice in the current bureaucratic and legal environments. They were under pressure to apply for Bhutan Medical and Health Council certification, though this was rarely enforced practically. Many feared that it was only a matter of time before their practices would be more rigorously controlled, if not banned outright. Such regulative tightening has been well documented elsewhere in the world (e.g. Ramsey 2009 on Canadian alternative practices or Saxer 2010 on Chinese-Tibetan medicine). Bodeker and Burford have argued that 'the global trend has shifted from being led by consumers and advocacy groups of practitioners, to a situation in most countries where governments are now working towards establishing a full regulatory context for the practice and use of [alternative practices]' (2007: 5). As they note, tighter regulation brings positive and negative outcomes to healers, patients and governments. Healers in neighbouring Tibet feel the pinch of bureaucracy, as documented by Diemberger (2005: 161):

> In the 1990s new policies that stressed standardisation within the country in the name of economic development had become increasingly prominent. A stricter control on local customs and on those phenomena that can be seen as superstition has increasingly been implemented. This can turn into a source of tension and legal inconsistency, so that local cadres find themselves unsure about how to handle phenomena which they used to tolerate as harmless parts of traditional life.[1]

Admittedly the context of Tibetan-Chinese relations differs from Bhutan, where such processes are only starting to occur. The tone was different in China, where 'economic development' was the goal. In Bhutan, the government prioritizes 'effective' and 'safe' healthcare for its citizens. The Ministry of Health views these 'parts of traditional life' as potentially harmful, especially if they use invasive procedures such as the cutting and sucking (*ra jip kyap ni*) administered to Pema, referred to in chapter 1.

As government regulations increased, there was a corresponding growth in litigiousness amongst patients and their families. Access to civil lawsuits and other such legal recourses was increasing. Healers had a growing fear of reprisal from patients, their families or those drawn inadvertently into the social waves of practice, as with Tandin who specialized in *ngan*. This type of defamation case follows section 317 of Bhutan's Penal Code (RGoB 2004: 43), which reads,

> A defendant shall be guilty of the offence of defamation, if the defendant intentionally causes damage to the reputation of another person or a legal person by communicating false or distorted information about that person's action, motive, character, or reputation.

Such legislation cuts directly into the social nexus of this healer's *ngan* practice, where blame and malicious intent can be ascribed to certain community members, amounting to what the law might see as 'defamation'. Suddenly healer malpractice lawsuits were becoming a possibility. Although this was not yet a common occurrence, the current trajectory indicated this might become so in the future. It is difficult to imagine such alternative practices continuing if such legislation gains greater traction. Iyer (2008: 94), in his article on defamation law in Bhutan, concludes by stating,

> For all the limitations of Bhutan's nascent legal infrastructure – including obvious constraints of judicial capacity – both the Thimphu District Court and the High Court have . . . made a promising, if imperfect, start which, on the whole, augurs well for the healthy development of defamation law in the future. Quite clearly, a number of crinkles need to be ironed out and a range of both conceptual and practical issues need to be clarified fairly quickly.

The legal challenges bearing down on Tandin and their conflict with *ngan* rituals was an example of what Iyer calls a practical 'crinkle'. While Iyer has an obvious agenda for a more rigorous legislative code, the 'crinkles' he mentions are more complicated in many of the everyday lives of patients and healers than he concludes. Within the narrative of this healer's pending lawsuit, the emotions of real people are involved. The patient suffered both physically and mentally from the anguish of being poisoned through magic. The healer feared legal reprisal and the loss of his livelihood. The accused neighbour was angry, perhaps for the first time exercising his defensiveness through a newly discovered legal right. While the gravity of the defamation law had not yet reached many healers, the process of 'ironing out the crinkles' in practices that carry with them this emotive social connectivity will surely be more complicated and nuanced than Iyer suggests, and it is unlikely to continue 'quickly' (Iyer 2008: 94). This will especially be the case given the public support for many alternative practices and their cosmologies. To certain limits, even the government supports them; 'customs' such as the belief and practices surrounding *ngag* or black magic are those that the government are hoping to 'preserve' with the culturally protective policies of GNH (see introduction).

Legal and bureaucratic pressures on alternative healers are increasing, and, in addition, patients themselves are calling for change. In chapters 1 and 2, I argued that patient demands on biomedical and traditional state healthcare practices were increasing. This demand was measured not only in patient or caseload numbers but also in requests for information, accountability, treatment quality and transparency from these services. I argued that such demand in the traditional-medicine services aided in the creation of a bio-traditional citizenship, whereby patients were identified by a *sowa rigpa* knowledge and practice that had its own nationalizing, standardizing and professionalizing agenda. It appears that a similar rise in the number of patient demands was occurring in the alternative practices. As a result of increased awareness of patient rights, service provider responsibilities and the possibility of legal action, healers met greater calls for accountability, professionalism and results. Although not true in all cases, I witnessed increased awareness around biomedical and traditional services that was starting to colour perceptions of alternative healers, changing them so that they were viewed as a type of non-institutionalized 'service'.

One case in point involved the Gopal family living in Mongar town centre, who wanted a *pawo* to perform a healing ritual for an ill relative. *Pawo* and *pamo* are spirit mediums, well accounted for in the literature on alternative healers in the whole Tibeto-Indian region (see T. Dorji 2007; Diemberger 2005; Pommaret 2009, among others). Diemberger (2005: 128) notes in her article on female oracles in Tibet that

> the titles 'pawo' (dpa '-bo) and 'pamo' (dpa '-mo), for men and women respectively, can be rendered as 'hero' and 'heroine'. They can refer to oracles as well as specific gods of a heroic nature and in some cases are connected to the bard-mediums who orate the Gesar epic. These terms are also used for mediums who embody other kinds of gods as well, and it is possible that the labels refer to perceived qualities of the individual medium.

These mediums are therefore active across the region with much variance in their practices, social positions and cosmological claims. While their 'qualities' (Diemberger 2005: 128) may vary from medium to medium, most *pawo* in Bhutan are possessed by deities, spirits, ghosts or the souls of the dead by means of intricately prepared rituals. The possessing entity often conveys messages or secrets to the living, perhaps revealing the perpetrator of the spirit's death, community members who are dabbling in black magic, harbourers of malevolence, reasons behind ill will or particular grudges and discontentments. During possession the *pawo* may convulse, lurch, speak in tongues and act erratically. I heard many stories where these frenetic possessions were cut with moments of extreme clarity, focus and intensity and messages from the possessor were communicated, sometimes in a language unknown by the *pawo* himself, often the mother tongue of the possessor (see T. Dorji 2007).

The Gopal family had determined that a spirit or ghost might be causing the illness of their loved one, and they hoped to address it head-on and cure the illness. Pommaret (2009: 130–31) notes this cause and response within a particular ethnographic example of the Gakha Dokha ritual in Trashigang, a *dzongkhag* east of Mongar, that requires one iteration of an intricate preparation:

> When people suffer from severe headaches, muscle pains, and body aches, if medicine does not cure them, people believe that this ailment is sent forth by the father and mother spirits. Therefore the Gakha Dokha ritual is commissioned. The process of the ritual begins with a vast display of offering items and varieties of colourful dresses hung on a frame tied to four poles erected in a 'c' shape. When all preparations are completed, the phrami (the name of a certain class of practitioners close to the pawo/ pamo) begins his ritual . . .

Unfortunately the Gopal family's ritual fell apart in the planning stages. The *pawo* had asked that the family prepare the foods, offerings, sacred objects, dress and incense. The family told the healer that they didn't know what was needed and that they expected him to provide these things; after all, they had commissioned him for the ritual. Communication faltered, and the night the healer and I arrived, there was nothing prepared. Conflict ensued. The healer expected the family to know what preparations were required and was angry at their ignorance of old traditions. The family resented the healer's lack of instructions and perceived apathetic performance, especially when they were paying him for his services. Ultimately both parties became fed up with each other, and the ritual was called off.

This narrative demonstrates how demands on and expectations of healers are changing, with patients and their families calling for greater accountability and responsibility from the healer as a 'service provider'. I would suggest that an increase in awareness and participation in the institutionalized forms of biomedical and traditional medicine, as well as the legal and civil rights granted to patients through these services, are affecting the expectations and behaviours of patients towards alternative healers.

There are other factors also playing a role in these changing perceptions. The calamity of errors in the Gopal family's story is set against a changing backdrop of how healers and patients work together and communicate. Most conversations, including the planning and negotiation of payment, can be done over mobile telephone, without the two parties meeting. Healers are often found by new patients through the sharing of mobile telephone numbers; these are networking tactics that alternative healers are fond of as they increase their caseloads. Yeshi, a very old, blind and partially deaf healer, carries a mobile phone so that patients can reach him. He can hardly understand what they say to him on the mobile, and vice versa, but he still values it as a new effective way to drum up business clientele.

Transport services are also getting better. However, this does not mean healers and patients are more likely to meet prior to a ritual or spend more time together. The opposite is true. Healers travel to a patient's home on the day of the ritual because they can. Previously the healer would have expected to travel to the patient's house and stay there a few days preparing and arranging the ritual in situ, a situation that may have prevented the conflict described earlier. Now this can be done from afar, and healers simply arrive at the time of the appointment or thereabouts; the joke 'We'll meet up at three PM BST (Bhutan Stretchable Time)' still rings true. The convenience of transport has thus compressed time rather than freed it.

It's important to note that the conflict between the *pawo* and the Gopal family was a single example where the ritual didn't work as intended. Every day many people successfully perform similar rituals to cure illness. The ways healers and communities operate is changing gradually, and many healers give ample time and attention to their patients.

One factor that holds these rituals together and propagates them in the face of mounting pressures is how they often involve networks of people rather than a simplistic one-to-one relationship between patient and healer. When a person falls ill, the entire household has to react and adapt. In farming families this is very pronounced because the loss of anyone to sickness also removes that person's labour from the equation. In urban settings, where routines of work, household chores and education typically take up much of the day, the illness of one family member can destabilize normalcy.[2] In such circumstances, especially in instances of chronic illness, relatives or community members might join the household to relieve the pressures surrounding patient care and daily activities. When families plan for alternative healers to visit the household, they rely on this wider network around the patient to work towards the cumulative success of the ritual and healing. This is especially effective in cases of illness that are rooted in disharmonious family or community relations. Family activities might include preparing particular foods, clothing, sacred objects or other religious paraphernalia. While the healer and patient will play key roles in the ritual itself, the familial care and community support for the household is also important to ensure proper hospitality and ritual functioning.

Economic exchanges among these surrounding social networks, especially between family members and the healers, also support the continuation of alternative practices. For one, they create an informal economy that helps support the livelihood of these healers. Tandin, embroiled in a lawsuit, made many complaints about the loss of his subsidiary income. However, economic or gift exchange also played a crucial role in the effectiveness of the practice itself. Take, for example, this story related by Yeshi to Singye and me while we visited his house in Mongar:

> There is an ancient story about a person falling sick and being unable to even move his hand. He was taken to a healer like me. The healer had refused to accept the money offered by the patient's family, and therefore the patient wasn't cured. Since the healer refused to accept the money, the patient's mother secretly hid some money underneath a banana leaf, with a *bang chung* [*bang cung*, traditional plates woven out of bamboo shreds] on top, and finally another banana leaf with some food on top. Because the healer refused the money, the mother offered the healer some packed

lunch but slyly made sure that the healer received the money by hiding it with the packed lunch.

On his way back, the healer came across the deity that had harmed the patient, disguised in human form. The deity then told the healer that he had received money, to which he replied that he hadn't received any, still not realizing that the patient's mother had slipped in the money along with the packed lunch. Though the healer was adamant that he hadn't received the money, the deity insisted that he had, and that because he had, the deity wouldn't be able to get any food, as he had lost the patient he was feeding on. The deity, in a fit of frenzy, fell off a nearby ridge. Later, when the healer reached his house and opened the packed lunch, he found the money.

Accepting money has become a norm since then. It was only after the realization that the healer had received the money that the patient showed signs of improvement; the patient was able to move his hand the next day, his leg the day after and on the third day the patient was on his feet, completely healed.

Without the exchange of money, the ritual and treatment was ineffective. Only when the financial exchange between family and healer was complete did the healing work. Note that this story emphasizes the requirement for the healer and family to consciously know that the exchange had taken place. Therefore, the visibility of the exchange is important, not just the exchange itself. The requirement for a visible or known exchange between healers and patient families helps to propagate the enactment of alternative practices along economic lines.

Social networks surrounding alternative practice also expand and become more complex between healers. I found that alternative practitioners would often work in tandem with other healers, oracles, astrologers or religious persons, amounting to an informal network of care providers. It can work similarly to a hospital setting where a patient visits first a diagnostician and then a specialist. If the specialist fails to cure the patient, they may send the patient to a different diagnostician or medical specialist. The same principles work for most alternative healers in Mongar. Astrologers, *lamas* and other religious individuals, either affiliated with a monastic institution or operating alone, often play the role of the diagnostician. These persons with divine powers identify the spiritual causation of a patient's illness. For example, in Mongar there are two dominant deities, one that lives on the eastern side of the town, the other residing below the sawmill on the western side. Each has its own territories, divinations and propitiations. The western deity even has a small house on a hillside that is cared for daily by a man employed by the local government; only he is permitted to enter. Religious insight is needed to identify which deity might have caused an illness, and which particular rituals would propitiate. Once the cause has been identified, the religious diagnostician sends the patient to a healer who specializes in the particular deity and ritual required. This often involves the healer knowing the deity's names and characteristics.

Yeshi described these healer networks and areas of expertise well. He specializes in the returning of lost souls, or as he calls it in Sharshop, *yong tsung ma*, literally translated as 'catching the fear' (*la tor, bla tor*).

I visit patients when they call me. Most of them are police wives and fathers. Usually they get better, especially those afflicted with 'fear'. But if someone is meant to die, how could they recover?

Sick persons [*nep, nad pa*] have to consult an oracle and the astrological charts to first discover what is making them sick. Sometimes they may also need to visit a *lama*. Whoever it is, they need to undergo a process of finding out what's wrong with them; this may mean checking urine and faeces, looking for colour variations. For example, if the bubbles in the urine are blue or black in colour, this means they have been poisoned [*dug*], possibly by a neighbour or someone who doesn't like them. If it's light or faded blue, then it's a case of a lost soul, usually by a malevolent spirit [*dü, bdud*]. I can't do these diagnoses. The sick person is referred to me only when the diagnosis is taken care of by someone else and it's a problem of a lost soul.

I have to tell the person's soul [*bla*] to come back. I first call out to the spirit [*dü*] by its name, the one who took the soul. I then call out the person's name. I do the 'introductions' [*ngo trö, ngo 'phrod*] between the person's soul and the spirit. I make ritual cakes [*torma*] and cake figurines [*lü, glud*] and offer them to the spirit. These are substitutes [*tsap ma, tshab ma*] for the sick person's soul. I shout out, 'Spirit! Your substitute has been given, now let him go! Lost soul! Come back!'

There is much more detail to this ritual. It includes the differences between deities and spirits, the relationship between Buddhist and non-Buddhist ideas of worldly deities and beyond-the-world deities, the types of poison, the methods of possession, the variations of illnesses or the expansion of ritual activities, but these complexities fall out of the purview of the current discussion (see Choden 2008 or Samuel 1993: 163–70, 176–98). Similar if not related practices are noted across the Himalayan region, with Nebesky-Wajkowitz (1956) offering some of the earliest ethnographic examples of rituals used to propitiate protective deities in Tibet. In the Bhutan context, T. Dorji (2004: 598–606) provides a valuable analysis of a similar healer's activities in Wangdue Phodrang *dzongkhag* in which he uses the Dzongkha term *sog* (*srog*), translated as 'vital principle' in place of the term 'lost soul'. Dorji (2004: 600–601) supports his analysis with his own ethnographic findings:

> Even in the towns among the literates, astrologers are still sought after for their advice especially in the case of prolonged illness or a failure of the medicines to improve the health of the one sick. At times the astrologer diagnoses the vital force of the sick person to have been severed by the srog gced class of malignant spirits. Indicating thus that the vital force has to be restored (srog blug). In consequence, the astrologer's first diagnosis is related to the identification of the problem with the prescription for solution. Based on the advice received from the astrologer, one of the relatives or neighbours of the sick approaches a medium for his assistance.

This practice of diagnosis and forwarding sick persons to religious persons, astrologers and healers amounts to an informal network of care providers. Within this network, the usual exchange of gifts, money, preference and amicable relations aid in the procurement of more patients, thus expanding a healer's income. Conversely, astrologers, oracles and religious persons, those acting as diagnosticians, also gain more patients from the recommendations of those treated by the healers. This cyclical feedback of patients within the network of alternative practitioners is vital to ensuring the continuation of their practices.

From the patient's perspective, this wider network and complication of aetiological variants helps to create a more 'holistic' enactment of their illnesses (Mol 2003). Again, as argued in chapter 1, cure, health and body multiplicity provide an agentive meaningfulness to patients. The cascading choices between alternative diagnosticians, the diagnoses themselves, and the healers that specialize in treating particular afflictions expand patient multiplicity and thus are valued by the patients that use them. However, the complexity of these networks and aetiological variants also requires a considerable amount of knowledge, social connection and navigation. Like in chapter 1 where I discussed patients collecting biomedical doctors' telephone numbers to secure access to hospital services, patients will collect, share and manage relationships with alternative healers. Therefore the effect on patients requiring the navigation of such healer networks is both a meaningful and taxing enactment of healthcare-seeking behaviour.

The networking between healers has received very little if any attention in literature on alternative healing in Bhutan, with exception of Choden (2008). Even the more ethnographic work such as T. Dorji (2004 and 2007) fails to address the importance of intra-healer relations and the ways this affects both the performance of rituals and the patients themselves. This is clearly a place for more research.

This section has tried to show how powers, pressures and demands in political, legal, social and economic discourses are changing the activities of alternative healers and the lives of the patients that use them. There is, of course, a sense of normalcy in many places and amongst many people, with such shifts going unnoticed. However, from the ethnographic vignettes provided here, I hope to show how these changes are slowly creeping into the everyday lives of these practitioners and patients. The future will undoubtedly bring further instances of conflict, resolution and adaptability to the ways that healers approach, communicate and interact with their patients, and vice versa.

Three Enactments of the Disease *Ja Né*

The wider social, political and economic contexts of alternative healer–patient relations have been explored in the previous section. I now zoom in to a specific, prevalent disease that was often referred to by patients, alternative healers, traditional medicine services, media outlets and the Royal Government of Bhutan. I focus on the ethnographic specificity of these disease enactments because, first, it grounds the wider network relations in the everyday experiences of patients; second, it helps explain how alternative practices engage with a complex patient multiplicity. Both of these discursive motivations fulfil the aim of this chapter: to understand how patients are affected by alternative practices. The disease explored is called *ja né*, and it has three different enactments that span biomedical, traditional and alternative practices. As I started to hear about this multifarious disease, I was at first confused as to what it was. The following story exemplifies the gravity and mystery of *ja né*.

A woman sat crying on a small wall outside Mongar Hospital's morgue. At ground level, stationed below the towering five floors of white concrete wall, she appeared small and lost. Her sobs were those of shock, as though her world had suddenly and radically changed. She also displayed a type of despairing fear, the kind associated with an implosion of life plans with little idea of how to cope and adapt to new circumstances. I walked up to her and asked if she was okay. The question immediately seemed redundant and insensitive.

A small taxi van with its back door open was backed up to the morgue's bay doors. From its rearview mirror hung the usual protective strings, charms and picture of a *lama*. A solar-powered plastic prayer wheel quietly spun on the dashboard. Huddled up in the back of the van lay a man's body swaddled by white cloth. The deceased was destined for his hometown where he would undergo his final rites and cremation. The driver was nowhere to be seen. Many taxi drivers refused to transport dead bodies, especially at night. Being so close to the dead and moving them across landscapes steeped in deities, spirits and ghosts was considered risky business by drivers and their customers. Ambulance drivers often displayed an air of incumbent practicality to circumnavigate these concerns. While this taxi driver had agreed to carry the body because of some familial relations with the deceased, he refused to be there during its loading. Out of sight, out of mind.

I was too uncomfortable – a telling sign of an ethical breach – to talk with the woman, and so I offered the little consolation I could and stepped away. When the driver returned to shower the taxi in purifying incense, he offered some more insight into the passing of his cousin. The man was only forty-five years old. He had contracted a quick and debilitating pain in his lower gut. I was told he had presented himself to hospital fairly promptly but the doctors were unable to cure his disease. Within a few days he was dead.

'What was the disease?' I asked.

'*Ja né*' he said.

Here it was again. *Ja né*. On moving to Mongar I had encountered this disease many times. Once I had identified it as an ethnographic subject it started appearing everywhere. It cropped up in interviews with alternative healers and patients, it was a topic of gossip, I heard it reported in the news and it was mentioned often in *drungtsho* consultations in the National Traditional Medicine Hospital in Thimphu and its nationwide units. This time it had taken a life. This was the most extreme and worrisome presentation in my fieldwork to date.

I needed more information about *ja né* in this particular case, and so I went to see the internal medicine physician of Mongar Hospital who had treated the deceased. He flippantly disregarded the idea of *ja né* as superstitious ignorance. He explained the man had died of a case of chronic liver failure due to alcoholism, a common diagnosis in Bhutan. Without any prospect of a liver transplant, there had been little hope for the man.

While this diagnosis was intimated to the man's wife and cousin, *ja né* was considered the primary cause of death. If *ja né* had killed this man, the disease was evidently serious. What was it? From my fieldwork I identified three variants of *ja né*, which manifested and were described in different patient contexts and healthcare discourses. This section explores these three types of *ja né* and how they span the biomedical, traditional and alternative treatment types. The different enactments (Mol 2003) of this disease show the complexity of presentation of apparently similar 'diseases' in patient's lives. Later in this chapter I present how a form of *ja né* was treated by an alternative healer, one of many conducting similar practices.

As I explain the three variations of *ja né*, it's important to note that the orthographic spelling of the term may change depending on its use. Dzongkha spellings, often dictated by the Dzongkha Development Commission, are different for the three variants, reflecting the distinctions of meaning. I have used the English phonetic '*ja né*' across all three variations of the disease because they were all pronounced the same by my informants. To help distinguish between them, I have added orthographic renderings using Wylie to highlight the difference in spelling. I have also attempted to analyze instances where these spelling variations tell of the different disease enactments.

First I begin with *ja né* as understood by traditional medicine. In one instance, a patient sat across from Singye, one of two *drungtsho*, in a consultation room in Mongar Hospital's traditional medicine unit. The patient offered his wrist to Singye for pulse analysis. He complained of unrelenting diarrhoea, fevers and headaches. He sat uncomfortably for a moment, sweating, as Singye gently pressed his fingers against the pulsing of his radial artery. Singye asked if he had travelled recently. The man replied affirmatively, saying that he had gone to India for a few days, just below the border crossing at Phuentsholing, to buy a car. The ongoing Indian rupee crisis, which was restricting foreign purchasing power, resulted in his empty-handed return (see Bisht 2012, Wangmo 2012 and *The Bhutanese* 2012 for more on rupee crisis), but he had spent some time there negotiating a sale. 'Ahhh, okay,' said Singye. 'You have *ja né* [*rgya nad*].'

How best to translate this traditional-medicine form of *ja né*? Singye, the *drungtsho*, spoke of a disease type familiar within the *sowa rigpa* canon. It even has a section in the newly released *Traditional Medicine Disease Classification* published by the National Traditional Medicine Hospital (2011: 191; see chapter 2). *Ja né* is associated with symptoms derived from changes in environment, climate or altitude, typically accompanied by changes in behaviour. Such changes commonly occur when travelling to different locations, such as the low-lying and hot lands of India or the mountainous regions of northern Bhutan.

Symptoms vary depending on the specifics of the locational changes. For example, travelling from low to high altitudes, common for many Bhutanese, results in such symptoms as headaches, light-headedness and giddiness, and along the continuum to severe and life-threatening altitude sickness. The full spectrum of these symptoms can be considered diseases of *ja né*. Likewise, a visit to the hotter climates of India, where cholera and typhoid are more prevalent, might result in *ja né*.

Behaviour changes concomitant with shifts of environment, climate and location are paramount in contributing to one's susceptibility to *ja né*. I discussed with Singye the case of the patient visiting India. Singye himself had just visited India and the border town of Phuentsholing to buy a car. He spoke at length about the behavioural risks associated with visiting the border areas with India. Drinking the different water was a major concern, particularly because of contaminants. There was also risk in eating rancid foods. While these are in some ways environmental factors, Singye saw his trip to India and the risks involved as behavioural changes. He had changed his diet and water habits, and these alterations to his normal routine exposed him to *ja né*. As he explained, other people on similar trips might also change their sexual behaviours, leading to *ja né*'s association with sexually transmitted diseases.

Diseases commonly associated with travel to Indian regions are well-known by *drungtsho* and patients who visit these places regularly, and they had a pronounced role in the history of Bhutan's relations with British India in the nineteenth century. The Duar Plains, a low, flat and fertile area of land south of the southern border mountains of Bhutan, were once inhabited by the Bhutanese population. In 1865, the British Indian government annexed these lands through a series of skirmishes, military operations and the Treaty of Sinchula (Singh 1978: 243), known as the Duar Wars (1864–65). This land later hosted India's largest and most profitable tea plantations. A running theme in some of the historical accounts written by Aris (1979), Aris and Davis (1982), Eden and Pemberton (1865) and White (1984) is the occurrence of malaria and other types of jungle-borne diseases during these five months of fighting. The hot and humid climate conducive to mosquitos, rancidification and infection resulted in significant loss of life on both sides. Such climate-risk notoriety has persisted in the traditional-medicine system, its teachings and in the patient populace of Bhutan. Those travelling to these northern Indian areas are commonly warned against the risks of malaria, waterborne diseases and other illnesses associated with heat and humidity. This first form of *ja né* as characterized in the traditional-medicine system thus has roots in such historiographies. These historical narratives in turn add an element of validation to such perceived risks.

Traditional-medicine *ja né* also takes into account patient behaviour changes regarding sexual activity, especially associated with visiting India. Singye noted that the pervasiveness of prostitution and unpaid sex in these border areas creates a risk of sexually transmitted diseases. While much of the blame for prostitution is put on the Indian side of the border, Phuentsholing too had a long-standing reputation as a beehive for brothels and paid-sex services. The *Kuensel* newspaper and other media outlets (*Bhutan Observer* 2012) have reported on the proliferation of such services and the arrest of prostitutes and 'pimps' (K. Dorji 2002). I met many people in Bhutan, especially men, who held the opinion that these Indian border towns play host to many brothels that are frequented by Bhutanese travellers to the regions. In Thimphu, some dance bars are also rumoured to host prostitution services, possibly influenced by these southern regions (Lorway et al. 2011). My research did not in any way extend to the validation of these claims, and I make no assertion of their validity. What is important to my ethnography is the connection between travel to these southern regions and changes in sexual activity, amounting to behaviour change associated with diseases of *ja né*. This is the first instance of sexually transmitted diseases entering the discourse of *ja né* symptoms, but not the last. As we will see, *ja né* and sex are closely connected in the third use of the term as deployed by alternative healers.

There is also an element of xenophobic prejudice that should be fleshed out in the use of the term *ja né* in relation to sexual conduct and visits to Indian provinces. The term for 'Indian' in Dzongkha is *ja gar* (*rgya gar*). While this is the official Dzongkha Development Commission word, its use in Mongar and in Thimphu, under certain circumstances, carries with it a negative and prejudiced connotation. The term *ja gar* might be spoken harshly, denoting a distain for the other, in this particular case an Indian person. This negative inference is similar to many other countries where national identities are opposed to neighbouring nationalities, constituting a juxtaposing 'otherness'. Shifting political and cultural identities surrounding national borders has had much attention in anthropology with Wilson and Donnan (1998), Gupta and Ferguson (1997) and Malkki (1992) offering in-depth analyses of power and culture between nation-states and the identities that define citizenship. Neighbouring nations have long attributed diseases to one another, with the historian Siena (2005: 12) noting how, during the Renaissance in the UK, syphilis was called 'the French disease'. Through the lens of such work, it becomes clear how prejudice can spread to disease classifications and their regional associations, as with this category of *ja né*. An example of this prejudicial leap is in the spelling of the terms. The connection and similarity between the *ja* in *ja né* and *ja gar* (*rgya nad* and *rgya ghar*, respectively) is telling of how concepts of the disease and its geographic aetiologies are related. This linguistic example parallels the historiographies of the nineteenth century, contemporary climatic and environmental risks and the change in sexual behaviours, all of which are associated with Bhutanese attitudes to their Indian neighbours.

Singye was a traditional medicine *drungtsho*, and this interpretation and use of the disease category *ja né* was firmly within the *sowa rigpa* canon. However, as seen earlier, some of the particulars of the disease, specifically the ways in which a person could become afflicted through travel and exposure to Indian border towns, takes on a more political, historical and cultural context. In this regard, I mean to make no association between such contemporary contexts and the tradition of *sowa rigpa*. The practice itself is separated and distinct from the examples of prejudice described earlier. *Sowa rigpa*'s understanding of *ja né* within its science of healing can stand apart from these socially contextualized occurrences, doing so in many other texts and medical institutions. I describe just some of the contemporary Bhutanese contexts that dictate how *ja né* as a disease of *sowa rigpa* is enacted and understood. Ultimately in the formal practice of Bhutanese traditional medicine, *ja né* is a disease related to changing environments and affiliated behaviours.

Now I turn to the second instance of *ja né* – a distinctive definition and enactment of the term, different from the one just described.

Late one evening I was sitting in Singye's house in central Mongar, helping his twelve-year-old son, Ugyen, with some science homework. While he puzzled over a question on volume displacement in a container of water, I reflected back on the days spent with Singye talking about the traditional medicine interpretation of *ja né*, the taxi driver's use of the term and various other instances of patient self-diagnosis. This was fairly early on in my identification of and investigation into the disease and its variations of enactment, and I was feeling particularly muddled. The directness and simplification of youth can often add clarity to complex ethnographic subjects like disease categories. Given that Ugyen's English was better than his father's – a realisation Singye was reluctant to admit – I decided to ask him what *ja né* meant in English.

UGYEN: You mean bird flu?
JONATHAN: Is that what it means in English?
UGYEN: Yes, *ja né*, it means bird flu, like the one on TV recently, in Chhuka.

He was referencing a news story on the Bhutan Broadcast Service in January 2012 (BBS 2012b) covering the outbreak, culling and containment of an avian influenza H5N1 event. On one evening I had happened to watch the footage of men dressed in white hazmat suits, goggles and face masks scurrying around dilapidated coops culling chickens and spraying the houses and nearby fields with disinfectant. Bird flu was a relatively new and unknown phenomenon in Bhutan, with the first outbreak recorded in 2010 in Rinchending, Phuentsholing (MoAF 2010). Reaction to these incidents by the National Incident Command Committee was swift, with many Bhutanese taking notice of this global disease phenomenon now hitting their national food chain. However, it should be noted that the 'Global Panic' surrounding avian flu, as described by Lockerbie and Herring (2009: 566–83), had not taken hold in Bhutan. Most people displayed little concern that it would affect their lives. But interest was piqued. Like HIV, credit cards and iPhones, international things new to the scene in Bhutan usually captured the curious mind, even if they were only partially understood.

Sensing the risk of epidemic, the government set to work on educating the population through television announcements, public health programming, town meetings and formal schooling. But, in 2010, it didn't yet have a Dzongkha name. The Dzongkha Development Commission – in charge of updating the Dzongkha language with current and new terminologies – assigned the term *ja né* (*bya nad*), where *ja* (*bya*) literally translates as 'bird' and *né* (*nad*) as 'illness' or 'sickness' (DDC 2012). The direct and uncomplicated association of the two simple and well-known terms gave bird flu national notoriety. Even this young boy, who spent most of his television hours glued to Manchester United football matches, watched the news, listened to his teachers and could recite the government-driven definition.

I asked Ugyen if *ja né* meant anything else. He said no. For him the meaning was singular, even though he may have heard his father, a *drungtsho*, use the term on a regular basis to refer to the traditional-medicine meaning of *ja né*. This highlights two points about the ways that diseases are understood, shared and interpreted in Bhutan.

The first is that diseases such as *ja né* can have multiple enactments. Recalling chapter 1's arguments regarding the patient multiple and Mol's (2003) work with the variations of the disease type atherosclerosis in a Dutch hospital setting, we see the potential for the multiplication of diseases, which in turn are enacted through patients' multiple healths and bodies. While father and son might discuss the *ja né* described on television, the father could expand the definition of 'bird flu' to incorporate elements of or differentiate from the *sowa rigpa* form of the disease. The disease categories can cross over, collapse and relate to one another. Bird flu could be a symptom of environmental change or incursions of foreign entities into new geographic areas by human or fowl. The recent outbreak was blamed on pigeons flying north from India (BBS 2012b) – again a 'southern' problem similar to the previous discussion of sexually transmitted diseases and India. Such intermingling of categories demonstrates how these two types of *ja né* exist in relation to one another and how they are enacted in different and similar ways. Given that the two terms are phonetically identical, slippage between the two meanings is common, creating the potential to collapse the terms or keep them distinctive.

The second point highlighted by Ugyen's singular understanding of *ja né* as bird flu speaks to the territorialization of biomedical assemblages asserted through government programming. His classroom, television programming, health activities and public health announcements are all avenues of communication for this interpretation of *ja né*. So powerful are these messages that Ugyen, whose father was a traditional *drungtsho*, did not encounter a variation of meaning. Ugyen also lived in Mongar town, where I met many alternative healers and their patients who used a third variation of *ja né*, to be discussed in the following paragraphs. These two communities in which he lived had not transmitted their enactments of *ja né*, at least in a way that impressed on him for recall. To give a measure of the power and pervasiveness of his educated understanding, Ugyen still did not expand his parameters of the term when he accompanied his father and me to visit a *ja né* healer regarding how to cure a form of the disease. While Singye talked with the healer, Ugyen and I discussed the issues of bird flu in great detail. Even in the face of other enactments of the disease, Ugyen's view of the bird flu variant stayed focused and centred. Therefore, the exploration of the variations of this disease category must include knowledge that the varying enactments can change in power and thus disperse into socialities of health and healthcare to varying degrees.

I have thus far described two forms of *ja né*, one used in traditional medicine, the other used by the government as a label for avian flu. Both have their own different official orthographic spellings, denoting their specific meaning within wider medical, historical, political and cultural contexts. One could also attribute the categories of traditional and biomedical medicine to these two enactments of the disease, highlighting the institutional and medical discourses in which they are distilled and propagated into patient communities. As yet, these two forms of *ja né* do not account for the disease that took the life of the man who was transported home in the taxi. To complete this cursory analysis of the full spectrum of *ja né*, I now introduce a third ethnographic subject of the disease, one more akin to the qualities, diversity and flexibility of alternative practices in Bhutan. This third form does not have an official spelling in Dzongkha, but would sometimes be noted in English as *bjaney* or *janey* in online publications (for example Tshering et al. 2013 and *Kuensel* 2013).

Singye and I continued our investigations into *ja né*, trying to meet as many alternative healers in the Mongar area as we could. One particularly hot day we found ourselves in a small town an hour away from Mongar, which hosted a massive hydroelectric dam, providing energy to India and income to Bhutan's coffers. Guarding this dam was a fifty-year-old man in a green military jumper, an army-issue beret and black boots. He took an hour off from his posting to perch on a wall and talk with us about his other job as an alternative healer. I will call him Tshering. Holding his rifle in one hand, leaving the other for animated gesturing, he told us of his healing practices and patient successes. He also offered a good starting explanation (in Sharshop[3]) of this third type of *ja né*:

> When somebody suffers from *ja né*, the symptoms of the illness are firstly pain in the navel area [*te wa*], and later the pain shifts towards the waist, lower back, and around the kidneys [*sha chi nang*] and to the back [*tshing khang*]. Lastly, there is no treatment when the pain reaches the neck [*ngang di ring*]. When the disease reaches the neck, there is no cure, and it pushes you out [meaning death]. Whether it's a man or a woman, the illness is the same. Even after treatment, if he or she dies, the disease will naturally come out from their genitals if it was originally *ja né*.

During my time in Mongar and in other areas of Bhutan, enactments of a third type of *ja né* were numerous, complex, sometimes disparate, but they often displayed a particular patterning, specifically in symptoms and treatment. I was told by many people that the popularity of this disease, meaning the frequency of its use in self-diagnoses as well as in alternative healers' diagnoses, had dramatically increased over the previous five to ten years. It had become a very real and present disease about which many people complained and to which they would respond by seeking out alternative practitioners who specialized in *ja né* healing techniques, like Tshering. These healers and their patients were also starting to appear in Bhutanese newspapers (Tshering et al. 2013) and online forums (*Kuensel* 2013).

Those suffering from this type of *ja né* often complain of pain from anywhere above the knees up to the middle of the torso. Pain sensations can include burning, itching, aching, throbbing, discomfort, stabbing or piercing in the upper legs, genitals, anus, buttocks, lower abdomen, kidneys, bladder or upper belly. Many of those suffering, both male and female, also mention genital discharge as well as pain while urinating and incontinence. Finally, some instances of *ja né* are accompanied by a loss of libido. This is a general list of symptom types and body locations that highlights the full spectrum of responses I encountered during fieldwork. However, some patients, doctors and healers would get more specific in their definitions, perhaps offering only one set of symptoms and afflicted areas to explain or define *ja né*. Pain and burning in the genitalia or bladder regions were the most common of these single-symptom explanations. Biomedical doctors would often translate this type of *ja né* into the biomedical disease 'urinary tract infection' according to its accompanying symptoms. Others I encountered also translated *ja né* into the gamut of sexually transmitted diseases, especially gonorrhoea, chlamydia, bacterial vaginosis, herpes and pelvic inflammatory disease. However, this was not always the case, as Tshering clearly noted when I asked if *ja né* were sexually transmitted diseases: 'No, it's not transmitted from having sex. Sexually transmitted diseases are like cancer or other diseases of these days.' What Tshering meant here was that sexually transmitted diseases are biomedical enactments, like cancer, liver disease or urinary tract infections. He was clearly drawing a line between these biomedical diseases and the *ja né* he treated. Ultimately I found that variance in the definitions of *ja né* were common, while some enactments were juxtaposed against others.

At this early stage of analysis, it's important not to compress the disease subject of *ja né* into these biomedical categories of interpretation, or any singularly defined disease alternative, as Tshering did in his rebuttal of *ja né* being synonymous with sexually transmitted diseases. Why? Firstly, this type of *ja né* exists for patients and healers as its own disease, without a biomedical interpretation. This *ja né* requires a particular form of cure, unavailable in biomedical and traditional practices. This again recalls chapter 1's discussions about multiple cures and healths. This *ja né* is its own disease and is not a part of the state-run biomedical or traditional medicine institutions. Patients in turn are created multiple in that they experience *ja né*–related diseases in all three of these enactments. Secondly, it would be premature to suggest that this form of *ja né* is only defined by problems relating to the genital and urinary regions. While this is by far the most common explanation for the disease, there are other symptoms and enactments of *ja né*. Consider these notes written by one of my translation assistants, who worked on similar research projects involving alternative healing practices, after listening to the recorded interview I conducted with Tshering:

> Sharshop Audio of Tshering with translation notes marked as '[TN]':
> I help patients with bone-setting [*tshig trug pa*] [TN: twisted nerves, fractured and dislocated bones of hands and legs], *dug toen ni* [TN: sucking poisons and impure blood], and when some illness occurs I do *me tsa* [TN: hot needle-piercing]. Also, I have to mention about a disease called *ja né* that I cure with my treatments . . .
> [TN: This is a type of disease but I'm not really aware of such diseases, and I don't know about *ja né*. Oh wait! I was told about a similar disease by a local healer called Jigme, sixty-one years old from Wangphu Village in Samdrup Jongkhar *dzongkhag*. He said that *ja né* was a type of malarial disease that happens mostly to women. The basic symptoms of *ja né* are red eye colouring and acting insane. The only treatment was sucking impure fluids from their genitals. But I'm not sure about what the healer sucks, either blood or pus.]

While there are some similarities emerging here, such as the relationship between *ja né* and the genital manifestation, this was not always the case. The narrative of the deceased man with a liver complication was another case in point. There was no evidence of sexually related diseases, urinary discomfort or genital pain; instead, only a stomach pain and eventually his fatality. The wife, the taxi-driver relative and the medical specialist confirmed that *ja né* was at least one interpretation of the disease. Therefore *ja né* and its symptoms spread wider than just urinary and genitally related problems and could incorporate other parts of the body and perhaps other knowledges and cultures about the body, health and illness.

What might cause this third form of *ja né*, and what might these aetiologies tell us about the disease itself? It was difficult to pin down an exact causation. For example, most healers when asked this question would say they weren't really sure. Tshering was a case in point:

'I couldn't track the cause of *ja né*. Until now I have assumed it might be caused by the air, the warm climate, or changes in temperature.' His response was similar to another healer, Nima, introduced later in this chapter, who denied knowing accurately the cause but suggested a few hunches, the most prominent of which was again change of weather or air temperatures. This is known in Sharshop to alternative healers as *tsed pa*, literally translated in the Dzongkha dictionary as 'malaria' (*tsad pa*, *tshad pa*) or more generally as 'fever'. This has direct linkages to the first form of *ja né* discussed in this section, where traditional medicine attributes causation to the change in environment or behaviour. Singye gave the good example of these types of change when visiting Bodhgaya, India, on pilgrimage. The term *tsed pa* may then include illnesses similar to typhoid, cholera, malaria, fever or diarrhoea.

However, concerning this similarity with the traditional medicine's form of *ja né*, this alternative form of *ja né* also includes poisons known as *dug*, as contracted through bad foods or water. This was corroborated in a recent *Kuensel* Online (Tshering et al. 2013) article that quoted an alternative healer from the Mongar *dzongkhag* as saying, 'Any person suffering from sudden illness is believed to have consumed or been given *dug* [*dug*, poison], for which sucking it out is the only cure.' This is not the same as *ngan* poisons, discussed earlier in the chapter, which have to do with ill-wishing or malevolent intentions from neighbours. Neither does it have to do with changing environments or behaviour. These are instead polluting elements that can cause *ja né*.

Finally, Nima and Tshering distinguished between sexually transmitted diseases and *ja né*, in particular that the latter could not be contracted through sexual intercourse. Sexually transmitted diseases (*lü drel né zhi, lus 'brel nad gzhi*) may show similar symptoms to *ja né* but are different, with the main distinguishing factor being the difference of transmission. To be more specific, one healer mentioned that sexually transmitted diseases come from outside the body, on contact with someone else who had the illness, whereas *ja né* originates from inside the patient's body. This is why they have to suck it out, to remove *ja né* from inside the body, a procedure graphically detailed in the following section.

This concludes my cursory analysis of the three types of *ja né* I encountered during my fieldwork. More research into these three enactments of the disease would undoubtedly shed more light on how they have come into popular illness discourses and continue to make their mark on patient experiences. I now focus on one instance of treatment. To further unpack the third form of *ja né*, the one discussed by Tshering the alternative healer, I turn now to how one healer treated this disease. Studying the actual practice of one type of *ja né* treatment can illuminate the effects of *ja né* on patients and the alternative healer community in Bhutan.

Sucking Genital Discharge

Having explored the wider contexts of alternative healers then zoomed in to a specific disease multiple identified by patients and alternative healers, as well as other institutional healthcare assemblages, I now focus on one iteration of *ja né* and how it was treated by an alternative healer. Through the examination of a healer's intricate practice and its growing popularity and pitfalls, we learn how patients in Bhutan are being affected by *ja né* alternative practices at the treatment level.

The third form of *ja né* is a real danger for many patients and healers across Bhutan, and especially in the Mongar region. It requires specialized treatment by a healer capable and experienced with the disease. I now introduce one such healer, who I call Nima.

I was sitting on Nima's floor for the second time in February 2011. My previous visit there with Singye had been fascinating, so we decided to return to ask more questions about this old man's healing practices. He offered us tea and later warmed up the beer I had brought as a gift, serving it hot like *ara*. I learnt on our last trip that his permanent home was a few hours east of Mongar, but he was happy to stay in temporary accommodation in the town for work reasons, and also because his wife and younger brother lived at home in a polyandrous marriage.

Nima corroborated the information from Tshering surrounding the risky progression of *ja né*. Both said that there are four stages of the disease, delineated by symptom severity and the number of days since onset. The first stage is characterized by a slow onset of pain and burning from the stomach, kidneys, lower back and genitals, typically within the first seven days of onset. Stage two sees an intensification of this pain and discomfort, along with genital discharge, common within twenty days. Stage three combines a worsening of the prior symptoms along with debilitating illness, including fevers, lethargy and malaise, within a month of onset. The fourth and most severe stage is unconsciousness or unresponsiveness due to the severity of symptoms, typically occurring after more than one month.

By stage three, Nima said that he was not able to cure the disease outright. He would perform his *ja né* healing practices but would then ask the patient or their minders to attend hospital immediately. By stage four any treatment was futile; as Tshering said, 'It pushes you out.'

Note that Nima encouraged his patients to visit hospital. Like almost all the alternative healers I spoke to, whether or not they specialized in *ja né*, they would often encourage patients to visit hospital. This marks a growing awareness amongst such healers about the curative services available from government institutions and suggests their willingness to collaborate with these services, at least on a referral basis. It also ties into chapter 3's argument regarding patients' use of multiple practices and their ability to incorporate patient multiplicity into their experiences of illness and healing. In following Nima's advice to visit hospital after his treatments, patients are again not deciding between practices but how to organize and order the use of multiple practices or illness responses.

Nima also mentioned that an important factor in being able to cure *ja né* is the speed at which patients seek out a healer. He said that waiting too long to seek treatment, i.e. a delay in healthcare-seeking behaviour, could result in symptoms worsening to stage three and resulting in incurability. Interestingly, this echoes similar concerns from many biomedical doctors and public health programming, as discussed in chapter 3. It appears that patient healthcare-seeking lag times and the resultant complications to diseases extends to alternative practices and their associated diseases as well. This adds further layers to the ethics, power and cultural complexity in trying to help patients choose certain services at appropriate junctures. If the patient arrived obviously displaying stages one or two of this disease, Nima would agree to perform his treatment. This would involve bringing the patient, either male or female, into his quarters and asking them about their pain experiences, including intensity, location and duration. He would also ask them if they were having any genital discharge. If they answered affirmatively, Nima would begin his procedure.

It begins with asking the patient to remove or rearrange their lower clothing so that their genitalia are exposed while in the supine position. At this time, family members or friends may or may not be present in the room, depending on the comfort of the patient. He then lights incense and recites *gnag* (*sngags*, mantra), offering protective words to ward off any malevolent spirits, ghosts or deities, as well as ill luck or ill wishes from community members. When afflicted with *ja né* and in this vulnerable position, with the body exposed undergoing a healing ritual, the patient is at a greater level of risk from such malevolent forces. Therefore *ngag* are a crucial protective part of the practice.

Once completed, Nima asks the patient to wash their own genitalia with warm soapy water. This is done to improve the hygiene of the general area and to remove any discharge that was exposed on surrounding areas. Nima also washes out his mouth, removing any substances or polluting materials.

Before continuing with his treatment, he also conducts a type of physical examination to confirm *ja né*. For a male he inspects the penis and looks for signs of retraction, where the penis recedes into the body. He also expects to see a yellowish or white curd-looking discharge from the urethra. He often touches the discharge, looking for the texture of curd. It may also feel similar to semen, but should identifiably not be. The penis head may also be red and uncomfortable. For a female, he looks for similar discharge. He also touches the patient's labia, looking for signs of physical change. According to Nima, if the labia flesh turns harder or softer on touch, this is a sign of *ja né*. It should be noted that this practice sounded erroneous to Singye – as he explained, tactile changes to the labia can occur due to the changes of blood flow to the region due to temperature change, touch, or a particular mental state such as embarrassment.

Once the examination is complete, he begins the treatment. He places his mouth against the genitalia of the patient and sucks the discharge out of the orifice. This is done with quick bursts of inhales rather than a prolonged slow inhale. Understanding the uniqueness, intensity and sensitivity surrounding this activity, I pressed Nima quite hard for specific details. I asked explicitly if the discharge enters his mouth. He said yes, this is unavoidable. Occasionally a small portion of the discharge might enter his throat to be swallowed; however, this is not intentional. Rather, he attempts to spit the fluids out, and he washes his mouth out with water so the fluids will not be ingested.

At this critical juncture in the description of this healing practice, I must be explicit in stating that I did not see Nima or any other healer conduct this practice. Given the sensitive and vulnerable position of the patients, only close relatives or friends join patients for the treatment. It would have been ethically inappropriate for me to attend a session. My data about Nima's practice, and that of Tshering and others, was derived from in-depth interviews and discussions with the healers, patients and many others claiming to have had the

treatment performed or known someone who had been a *ja né* patient. I present
this practice here as valid ethnographic evidence on the grounds of repeated
corroboration by many of my informants of Nima's account of his practice. As
a rigorous and occasionally sceptical researcher, I ensured that the information
presented to me by Nima was corroborated and validated by many other people,
across diverse professional, gender and age ranges.

When analyzing this practice it is important to distinguish it from other
types of 'sucking' healing practices, well documented in anthropological literature. Nima's intention is to remove the discharge from the patient, not for him
to hold the fluids himself. His body and mouth are simply the physical tools that
do the best job. Additionally, the fluids are seen as polluting elements rather
than a spirit or other type of non-material agency. This is very different, say, to
the practices of African shamans among the Ndembu people, written about
extensively by Edith Turner (2011), who remove both an 'afflicting spirit' and a
'human concrete tooth' (165). Her work is connected with her late husband
Victor Turner (1957, 1962 and 1967) and Michael Harner (1980), who both conducted fieldwork with shamans who were 'aware of two realities' (Harner 1980:
116). These complementary works delve into the analytical and ethnographic
complexities of sucking practices where both physical objects and metaphysical
spirits are removed from patients' bodies. Edith Turner notes the replication of
such dualistic spirit-physical worlds through other ethnographic work such as
Cawte (1974), who wrote about doctors in the Waliri of Australia who found a
'dingo spirit inside a patient which they extracted in the form of a worm' (Cawte
1974: 48, qtd. in Turner 2011: 165). These practices and countless more from the
bookshelves of similar ethnographic projects describe instances where healers
suck some form of a spirit or metaphysical subject out of the patient. Nima
explained to me that this is not the case in his practice. Instead, he removes
poison known as *dug* which causes the *ja né* illness. This poison presents itself
as a polluting fluid, the discharge, or as he sometimes calls it, *né* (*nad*, meaning
disease or illness). While religious and spiritual cosmologies are inherently
attached to the patient's illness and health, this practice appears to be, for Nima,
one of removing polluting materials rather than spiritual agents.

This does not, however, rule out the importance of spiritual and religious
powers for other aspects of the *ja né* removal. Nima is aware that sucking
genital discharge brings with it risks of illness for him. He is concerned that he
might get *ja né* by accidentally ingesting the fluids and *dug*. This is why he
cleans out his mouth and the patient's genitalia with water before continuing.
But he also said, 'If by accident gulps of fluid go down my throat, nothing wrong
happens. This is because we have *gnag*' (*sngags*, mantra). In reciting mantra
before and after the sucking, he calls upon a religious power to protect him
from contracting *ja né*. Therefore he brings in a spiritual method of protection
against the polluting fluids.

While Nima uses his mouth, other healers told me of other methods to
remove the discharge. Tshering discussed his methods for curing *ja né*:

Previously we used a bamboo pipe to suck it out. But nowadays we use a hospital pipe [syringe] or a big pipe [syringe] from the livestock hospital instead. If we use a hospital pipe, we don't have to suck by mouth. But we also must recite mantra while extracting, or else it doesn't work.

The adaption of biomedical health tools is becoming more common amongst alternative healers. In this instance of *ja né*, the practice of discharge extraction can be performed by mouth or with a similar vacuum-creating implement. This does not detract from the practice's efficacy, highlighting that the removal of discharge is a physical manipulation of a patient's body, similar to setting a broken leg. However, Tshering was quick to point out that mantra is also required, therefore emphasizing a dimension of the practice not included in the physical removal of body fluid. This fortifies the spiritual elements of the practice.

Adaption to biomedical equipment extends beyond *ja né* and into other popular alternative healing practices, such as the cutting-and-sucking practice used by Pema in chapter 1. Again Tshering added valuable insight into how healers are adapting this practice with the arrival of new equipment: 'While cutting, we use sterilized blades as we find in hospitals. We use these blades to make three small cuts, not big. Then we suck out the impure blood by using a ram's horn [*lug ra, lug rwa*].'

Tshering uses sterilized blades from hospitals, often acquired through hospital contacts or other non-direct means. The hospitals and BHUs I visited did not proactively give out sterilized blades, generally disapproving of the practice due to the risk of infection. This disapproval transferred to alternative healers who are increasingly aware of the risks of using unsterilized blades in such practices. Patients and doctors, both biomedical and traditional, increasingly demand that blades be sterilized. While Tshering employs sterilization techniques, they are relatively new, and are most likely used sporadically at best by healers across Bhutan.

While the blades in this cutting-and-sucking practice are traditionally home-made, new hospital blades are being used to the same effect. Similarly a switch from mouth to syringe (*men khap, sman khab*) tools is occurring for *ja né* healers without adversely affecting the practice. However, not all implements could be changed due to certain healing qualities of the materials. Tshering made a note of this as he discussed the type of horn used in the cutting and sucking:

To suck the impure blood, we need a ram's horn [*lug ra*]. If unavailable, we cannot use just any animal's horns. We can use the horn of a wild goat [*jag ra, byag ra*], and if it is not available then we use the white horn of a *ja tsha* [*rgya tsha*, cattle crossbreed]. If we were in Marak and Sak Teng [eastern Bhutan regions], we could use the horn of a *drang lang* [*drang glang*, ox crossbreed].

The particularity of animal horn required for cutting and sucking is an important example of how such tools are specific and non-substitutable with biomedical alternatives. However, this rigidity is also changing. Although these guidelines dictated Tshering's practices, I heard other healers claim they used syringes for producing the vacuum during cutting and sucking. Public health initiatives, the growing scarcity of these animal horns and the demands for greater health safety from patients are some of the factors driving these changes.

Without replacement tools, Nima willingly uses his mouth to remove genital discharge. This raw form of the practice was well known to many of my informants in the Mongar region. An ambulance driver I spent a few days with while racing around Mongar roads described this exact practice when I asked him about *ja né*. His facial expressions clearly reflected his queasiness at the thought of Nima's practice, but he accepted it as a well-used and well-known practice in everyday life in Mongar. He is not alone in his dubious yet accepting reaction. Many patients opt for this *ja né* healing practice, and it is gaining national prominence, for both positive and negative reasons, the latter well-exemplified by an article in the *Bhutan Today* newspaper on 14 September 2011 (Dema 2011):

> The Thimphu district court convicted a forty-three-year-old man from Dramitse gewog under Mongar Dzongkhag to five years of imprisonment on August 31, for raping a 19-year-old student.
>
> The judgment was passed by bench III of the Thimphu district court. He will be serving time from August 1, 2011 to August 1, 2016.
>
> The convict is a former army personnel. The victim and her mother had gone to visit the convict in Lungtenphu last July as she was suffering from a pain in the leg. The accused had asked the mother to wait outside and took the girl inside a room. He then asked the girl to undress after which he molested the girl. The convict had asked the victim not to tell anyone about the session.

A missing specific in the article is that the man was a healer and had attempted to convince the young girl that sexual intercourse would cure her ailment, a detail added in a *Bhutan Observer* (2011) article. This case was deeply concerning for most people who followed it across national newspapers. It spoke to the central concern of many regarding such *ja né* healing practices, that they are instead sexually motivated. It also showed the potential for sexual motivations to be hidden behind a guise of faux treatment. Similar cases have been reported where alternative healers prescribe sexual intercourse to cure *ja né*. Often *ja né* was reported in these cases as a urinary tract infection (see *Bhutan Observer* 2011). Ultimately, this healer and many others were accused of using their sometimes highly regarded position as 'sacred healer' for malicious or sexual ends.

A few *Kuensel* Online forum (2013) entries from 2011 convey the negative sentiments surrounding this case in an anonymously direct fashion (grammar edited):

> POSTING 1: Yes, the traditional healers have healed themselves of their urge for lust by tricking sick girls/women that approach them for help. . . . The multiple cases of adultery and sexual activities with sick people prove them as liars that need to be punished for doing contrary to what they were understood to be doing.

POSTING 2: You and I should have no faith in them . . . stop going to them . . .

POSTING 3: I was already having doubts when I first saw healers do these things under locked door. Moreover, they claim most women and girls are suffering from janey [*sic*]. I feel we should be careful when they claim such disease for treatment.

But not all posters shared these negative outlooks:

POSTING 4: Although many have misused the traditional method of healing janey [*sic*], there are some genuine healers who have healed many in the absence of modern-day medical services. So we need to really look at the genuineness. Not all healers are rapists.

This brings us back to Nima and why patients were still visiting him, even after the conviction of the healer from Dramitsc. *Ja né* was considered a real and dangerous disease that in most cases required the healing practices of an alternative practitioner like Nima. As Tshering told me, 'There are no treatments for it in hospitals.' While the Ministry of Health, biomedical doctors and traditional *drungtsho* would undoubtedly refute this statement, it appears many patients in Bhutan believed it to be true, and continued to visit Nima or other *ja né* healers.

The influence of *ja né* on patients and their families, and the importance of Nima's intervention, was best illustrated by a story corroborated by a number of hospital staff. A male patient lay critical and unconscious in an unnamed intensive care unit, engulfed by oxygen pipes, beeping machines and twenty-four-hour supervision. Only two family members at a time were allowed to his bedside and were only permitted to use the provided slip-on shoes at the unit's doorway. This level of supervision and restriction was unlike any other part of the hospital except for the surgical theatres that barred any from attending. Late one evening, when the doctor was at home sleeping, the patient's family pleaded to the night nurse to permit a *ja né* healer into the ward to conduct the genital discharge sucking practice. She eventually relented, and the healer snuck in and conducted his healing practice on the unconscious patient right there in the ward, including the sucking of genital discharge. The nurse kept this from the doctor, but news spread, and he soon discovered what had happened. He was furious and reprimanded the nurse. The act was considered an invasion or incursion by this healer into a space in which he had no right to be. With the intensive care unit being the epicentre of Bhutan's biomedical offerings given the technology, investment and care offered in its secluded ward, it was unacceptable that an alternative practitioner be permitted to practice there.

Biomedical doctors will often give patients space to decide if they wish to visit an alternative healer, even though they may frown on their practices. They leave the ultimate decision-making up to the patient and respect their agency. However, in this case, the healer was on their turf, which was inexcusable. While politeness, respect and political correctness can often blur the lines of acceptability between alternative and biomedical practices, this injunction clearly denoted the void between this doctor and the healer. In my work, never was the unacceptability of alternative practices more clear than in the opinions of that doctor whose ICU patient was visited by a *ja né* healer.

While the doctor propounded these opinions, it was the patient's family who chose to employ the healer. After all, they were the ones who persuaded the night nurse to permit him into the ward and, taking responsibility for the unconscious patient, were there to make decisions for him. Thus, while biomedical doctors and traditional *drungtsho*, as well as Ministry of Health public health policy, oppose *ja né* healing practices, patient demand remains high and evidently cunning.

While this section has focused on Nima's and Tshering's *ja né* healing practices primarily in the Mongar town, there is growing evidence that *ja né* healing is also popular in the surrounding Mongar *dzongkhag*. I quoted in chapter 1 a *Kuensel* Online (Pelden 2012b) article that stated there were 1,683 alternative healers in Bhutan, 100 of which were in Mongar *dzongkhag*. Although details of what these alternative healers offer were omitted, continuing Bhutanese journalism seems to be providing a growing amount of interesting data. An August 2013 *Kuensel* Online cover story (Tshering et al. 2013) entitled 'Traditional Healers: Quacks or Miracle Curers?' identifies the growth of specifically *ja né* healers in the Mongar region, quoting one: 'People rely on us to treat bjaney, where healers suck out poison from the genitals.' Later the article claims that 'in Mongar, there are at least two or three traditional healers in every village.' The regional use of alternative healers, including those performing *ja né*, is being made more evident by such journalism, adding important ethnographic data to what is a widely known yet under-published alternative practice. More detailed ethnographic research as well as more comparative studies in Mongar and other *dzongkhags* would yield more information about frequency of use and patterning between the illnesses and curative practices surrounding *ja né*.

Conclusion: Appropriate Practices?

This chapter has charted three scales of alternative practice in Bhutan. At its widest gaze, it explored some of the political, social and cultural influences that affect alternative practices and, as a result, the patients that use them. The chapter then narrowed into an alternative disease phenomenon known as *ja né* and how it has multiples of meaning or enactment. Narrowing further, the final section took one of these enactments of *ja né* and described in ethnographic detail how it was treated by a Mongar alternative healer. In doing so, we saw some of the contentions arising from such practices alongside a steadfast patient demand.

The discussion and explanations of the alternative form of *ja né* requiring genital discharge removal has focused on the specific ethnographic examples that I encountered in Mongar. The healers I worked with had specific explanations for *ja né* and how it should be treated. They noted the role of *dug* (poison) in causing *ja né* as well as its corresponding symptoms, including genital discharge. They also explained a strict weekly progression of the illness, ultimately resulting in death. But patient explanations of symptoms and causation surrounding *ja né* extended beyond these healer's interpretations, and included a whole range of symptoms and cross-infection possibilities. The widow's claim that *ja né* caused her late husband's death or the risk of contracting *ja né* through sexual intercourse were two examples examined here. This highlights the important point that *ja né* is in many ways a transmutable and changeable disease category for those who use it to enact their illnesses. While it was often linked to physical symptoms, it retains a social flexibility and can be used to describe any number of health issues.

This disease flexibility is important when considering other occurrences of *ja né* in different fieldsites in Bhutan. It is very likely that further studies on this disease would reveal further complexity. Any future research should take into account the performative diversity of *ja né* and the important role this variability plays in the agency and meaning of the disease for patients and healers.

Alternative practices, such as the few described here, reveal important and challenging questions regarding the 'appropriateness' and 'safety' of procedures like the sucking of genital discharge and cutting and sucking. Although I never heard of a *ja né* or cutting-and-sucking healer complain of cross-contamination, the risks are obvious. The health risks associated with alternative practices are well known to the Ministry of Health, which asserts the strong message that practices like genital discharge sucking are neither appropriate nor safe.

It is vital to understand that not all alternative practices carry with them the weight, severity, risk, contentiousness or invasiveness of the *ja né* practices described in this chapter. Many alternative healers treat patients without negative pressures from media or the Ministry of Health. Schrempf (2015a) cites a good example of an alternative healer conducting a lost-soul-retrieval practice who avoids many of the challenges and risk analysis being posed by the Ministry of Health. The removal of *ja né* as described here stands as an extreme example of alternative practices questioned by media, the Ministry of Health and many healthcare professionals, as well as patients. But it is important to keep in mind that not all alternative practices carry this controversy. With the huge diversity of alternative practices in Bhutan, many are safe, complementary to the institutionalized healthcare offerings and valued by the patients that use them.

Thus far I have attempted to maintain a levelled neutrality in analyzing the practices surrounding *ja né* removal and other alternative practices, preferring to describe the actions of healers, patients and doctors as I met them, as well as some of the wider social contexts in which these practices took place. I have also attempted to highlight how such alternative practices affect patients. I concluded to this end that patients were visiting these healers regularly, and gaining agentive meaningfulness in engaging with these practices. Having returned from the field and discussed these practices with many outside of Bhutan, I have often been asked, 'Did these alternative practices work?' This question deserves an answer.

I met many people and healers who professed that these practices do help patients. They would often claim that the sucking practice would, could and did cure *ja né*. Patients engaging with this practice, except for those who were or might have been sexually assaulted, found the treatment efficacious. Certainly they found meaning in the practice inasmuch as they felt the occurrence of healing. This experience of healing in the enactment of the genital discharge sucking practice was important to patients in curing their *ja né*, and if you asked them, they would tell you, as they did me, that yes, it does work.

However, if genital discharge sucking does cure *ja né*, it might not be effective in treating other symptoms that may or may not be related to the *ja né* disease itself, such as the biomedical defined symptoms of a urinary tract infection. For example, many patients would visit the hospital after being treated by Nima; he would often direct them to do so. Without alerting the doctors in Mongar Hospital of the practice they had engaged, patients would take a course of antibiotics or other medication and enjoy the symptomatic relief that it would bring. This way both the urinary tract infection and the *ja né* were present, treated and cured. Again I recall chapter 1's argument regarding the multiplicity of healths, which claimed that patients have many sides of their health that could fall ill and ameliorate in different ways. Sometimes, as possibly in the case of *ja né* and a urinary tract infection, both diseases present with the same symptoms, although the enactments of health are different. Thus two treatments are required, both of which bring meaningfulness to the experiences of suffering and healing for the patient.

This is an analytical argument, not an ethical one. It also opens the potential for diseases like *ja né* to exist in the socialities of health and healthcare in Bhutan without asserting a medical agenda onto the practices and diseases themselves. It was a goal of this chapter to let the ethnographic actualities of *ja né*, its healers, patients and pundits to exist without scepticism or pre-emptive judgement.

This does not, however, deny the tensions between these enactments of diseases, the practices to heal them and the practitioners themselves. I tried to show in the case of the sexual assault and the negative public response that such multiples of health and cures are hotly contested on a daily basis. And for good reasons. The Ministry of Health, its biomedical doctors and many of the traditional medicine staff – i.e. the institutions of medical practice in Bhutan – strongly oppose such practices due to, among other things, the perceived health and safety risks ascribed to them, vulnerability to assault, delay in healthcare-seeking behaviour, symptom aggravation, infection and misdiagnosis. The ethical, safety and moral boundaries are clear in practices as extreme as genital discharge sucking: it is not accepted and should be discouraged if not eradicated completely. This stance is meant to protect patients from further suffering and in many cases has helped patients whose symptoms were not alleviated through alternative practices.

The goal of this chapter has not been to undermine these efforts and ethics of the Ministry of Health, but to describe healing practices as I encountered them in the field, among the patients and practitioners who used them. It is my hope that those interested in the betterment of the health of Bhutanese patients can use this chapter to learn about some of the current and actual practices of healing, while offering potential avenues of constructive engagement with both healers and patients.

Notes

1. In the same article Diemberger (2005: 150–55) lists another example of bureaucratic control, but this time by the Tibetan government over oracles' practices in the 1920s and 1930s. The issue of regulation is therefore not a modern phenomenon but has instead been a regular activity of institutions and bureaucracies overseeing healthcare-related activities.
2. See Wikan and Barth (2011: 13–23) for more on family structure.
3. Given that Sharshop has no written language, I have excluded orthographic spellings in the quotation.

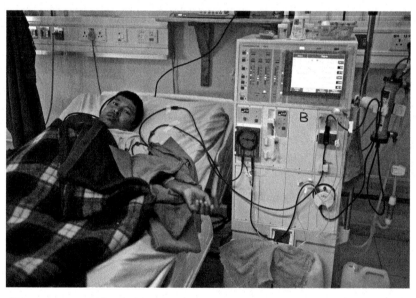

Illustration 5.1 Blood Flows through Humans and Machines, *Mongar Hospital, Mongar.* This patient visits the dialysis ward three times a week. He moved his entire life to Mongar to use this machine. Given the speciality of the equipment, the ward is private, permitting only patients and a single accompanying family member, although this patient came alone. His family didn't move with him to Mongar.

5

Patients and Healing Materials
Relations and Dependency

Introducing Material-Patient Relations

In an isolated dialysis ward in Mongar Hospital, a hollow needle pierced a man's median cubital vein. Blood flowed from his vein into a hemodialysis machine, where it was pumped around a circuit and through a semipermeable membrane. From there it counter-flowed against a fluid called dialysate, which removes high concentrations of urea and creatinine. With its chemical constituents rebalanced, the blood was returned to the man's body through an inlet needle near the outlet.

Two floors below, a traditional-medicine patient suffering from an aggravated wind (*lung*) humour disorder was handed a small plastic bag of pills scribbled with a few symbols denoting ingestion instructions. Unable to read, the patient opened the plastic clasp and gobbled down some of the round pills. They crushed against his teeth and settled in his belly. The pills had been tested in a dissolution bath in the Menjong Sorig Pharmaceuticals factory in Thimphu; the thirty-six-herb concoction would take four hours to dissolve fully and enter his bloodstream. These thirty-six herbal agents would react with this man's karmic constitution in over a million different relations of chemicals, compounds and humoral qualities. There could even be a placebo effect; the *drungtsho* was aware of this and hoped it would occur, thus increasing all-round efficacy. The man slipped the remainder of the pills into the fold of his *gho*, smiled, and walked out.

Later, while walking between wards, I passed a *gomchen* (lay monk), swathed in his maroon and purple robes, sitting in a wheelchair that was made in India. A crumpled brown paper bag on the monk's lap contained a spaghetti web of protective colourful strings (*sung kü, srung skud*) and paper amulets (*sung ma, srung ma*). He offered one to me for five *ngultrum* and I accepted: I needed some good luck for my upcoming three-day car ride back to Thimphu. An hour later I saw him in the maternity ward, wheeling around the ten beds filled with hot and uncomfortable pregnant mothers-to-be. Business was good. He handed out handfuls of these strings that had been blessed by a high *lama*, which the women draped across their bellies and necklines. The friction of the synthetic polyester strands against bare belly skin brought calm to the mothers. The room fell silent. Audible only were a few deep breaths and the rattle of the chair wheels as the monk glided down the corridor looking for his next sale.

Patients are constantly and unrelentingly encountering healing materials. When they become patients – in other words, when they fall ill and form a relationship with something or someone that offers treatment of their illness – they ineluctably connect to materials of healing. To a patient, everything becomes a material of amelioration or harm. Illness itself is a perspective of the world and its materiality, investing common objects with new and personal meaning. An eighteen-year-old eyes a steep dirt track up to a mountaintop house very differently from an elderly sufferer of chronic arthritis. A healthy nose smells a hot cup of *ara* differently than the nose of a person with liver disease. A body in pain, near death, may find less comfort in a morphine injection than in the touch of a hand deemed sacred due to centuries of reincarnation. Through illness and the processes of patient emergence, materials transform. In turn, transformed materials affect patients.

This chapter will focus on a specific type of healing materials – biomedical pharmaceuticals – and their concurrent effects on patients. I will argue that healing materials in Bhutan have undergone radical changes over the past decade (McKay 2007; Melgaard and Dorji 2012). Patients are now faced with new materials in traditional, biomedical and alternative healing, many of which have been adapted to increasing regulation, institutionalization and service centralization. Included in my use of the term 'healing materials' are the medicines, technologies, machines, surfaces, bodies or any other types of 'objects' that patients interact with to promote healing. As seen earlier, a dialysis machine, a complex herbal medication or a piece of sacred string could all fit within this definition.

New types of material influence the ways patients experience suffering and healing and also often define the parameters of decision-making. This latter point connects this chapter to the central theme of this book: patient healthcare-seeking behaviour. It will show that healing materials play a defining role in the practices, healths and bodies that constitute the patient multiple. Therefore material-patient relations are central to healthcare decision-making processes and the ways that patients assemble, manage and navigate their patient multiplicity.

How are these material-objects connected to patient-subjects? Borrowing from Bruno Latour's Actor Network Theory (2005 and 1987), specifically his engagement of non-human actors, I argue that materials are load-bearing agencies, affecting both other non-humans and social worlds. As Miller notes in his introduction to materiality, Latour 'emphasises the agency of this non-human world such as microbes or machines, which cannot be reduced to a mere epiphenomenon of the social' (2005: 12). Miller stresses Latour's insistence on the power and agency of non-humans within social networks. 'Objects' therefore become 'subjects' that have meaningful effect on the world. In the framework of my research, patients' worlds – their phenomenologies, socialities and understanding of suffering and healing – are partially constituted by these affecting material-subjects, as demonstrated in the earlier ethnographic vignettes. This chapter seeks to understand how these materials exert agentive power across political, social and economic networks and consequently affect patients' experiences of suffering and healing.

The central section of this chapter looks at the changing scenario of biomedical pharmaceuticals in Bhutan and how change affects patients. The analysis involves a close examination of patient-material relations. The ethnography presented concerns the increase of different drug types and their availability through national hospitals, health clinics and retail pharmacy shops. At the time of my fieldwork, the country was undergoing what was called a 'national drug shortage', where changes in drug regulation policy inadvertently created a bottleneck of supply. The reaction of doctors, patients and the media was pronounced and intense, indicating the power and place these drugs had in the health socialities of Bhutan. To demonstrate this new landscape of pharmaceutical agency and how it affects patients, I use an ethnographic story of tragedy: Neyzang, a female patient suffering from chronic heart disease, died in Mongar. The cause of her death was contested by many interlocutors, but one important possible reason was a lack of medication. This section will not attempt to settle this issue, but it will explore how the discourses, lines of reasoning and claimants enmeshed in this tragedy reveal the reality of patient-material relations in Bhutan. Patients must adjust to a complex new medical materiality operating on both a local and global scale.

I conclude by returning to the central theme of this book, patient healthcare-seeking behaviour, and asking how this might be affected by the forms of healing materiality. I assert a potential practical application for materiality by the Ministry of Health and its healthcare institutions. My findings will show that patients are increasingly attracted to curative materials that have a particular effectual quality or allure. I argue that the Ministry of Health could present the materials of both biomedicine and traditional medicine in such a manner as to further encourage appropriate first-response healthcare-seeking behaviours. I also assert that education for patients and advertising in respect of specific material availability in national healthcare centres could have a strong effect on the decisions patients make about the timing of their first visit to hospital.

While the subject of biomedical pharmaceuticals is focused on my fieldsite in Mongar, it is informed by networks and powers way beyond the scope of everyday interactions between patients and materials. Biomedical materials are engaged and constituted by international and national discourses of trade, ethics, economics, regulation and science. Therefore, the ethnographic vignettes of patient experiences and material narratives will also be explored in this wide contextual frame. To these ends, volumes such as *Global Pharmaceuticals:*

Ethics, Markets, Practices by Petryna et al. (2006) provide important starting points for what these international discourses are and how they have power over patients' lives in places like Mongar and Thimphu. I will draw from this volume throughout this chapter.

Following the themes of the previous four chapters, this final one looks at the biomedical assemblage of healing. This chapter examines specific forms of materiality within this assemblage and how this materiality engages with end consumers. To focus the ethnography and analysis, I have omitted an exploration of materials used primarily in the traditional and alternative practices. I have chosen to focus on biomedical materials here partly because of the dearth of publications in this area. The variance and application of materials in the alternative practices has had some attention, as discussed by T. Dorji (2004, 2007, 2009), Tempa (2011) and Pelgen (2000). Another reason for my focus is that the changes in biomedical materiality are happening fast and exponentially. This recent growth means that patients are increasingly incorporating these materials into their experiences of suffering and healing, and they are poised to do so further. Focus on biomedical materiality now could empower healthcare providers to better manage patient-material relations in years to come.

Pharmaceuticals and the Changing Materialities of Patient Demand

On a winding road between the small village of Khaling and Mongar, in a tiny silver Alto car, Neyzang's heart stopped. Moments earlier she was cradled in her father's arms, coughing up blood, struggling to breathe as fluid filled her lungs. Blood replaced oxygen, suffusing her vacuous cavities. Unable to breathe, she died at thirty miles per hour, only ten miles from Mongar Hospital.

Later that day and unaware of the tragedy besetting a grieving family, I ran into a contact of mine, a journalist for the *Kuensel* newspaper, who was stationed to cover local Mongar news. That afternoon he uncharacteristically sagged in his chair, his torso and face appeared sombre and melancholy, while his fingers impatiently thumbed a ballpoint pen. I asked if he was feeling sad. He said he was but then fell quiet. We sat in silence together, I pondering his emotional state, he considering my trustworthiness. A few moments later he leaned in close and in a hushed voice said that his cousin had died that morning, a twenty-two-year-old mother of one, on the way to hospital. It was because of drug shortages, he said. He was going to write an article about it and blow the story wide open.

In some ways his account was not new. The saga of Bhutan's pharmaceutical drug shortages began somewhere in 2010 and had received constant national news coverage, with the most recent stories citing the rupee crisis as an additional layer of complexity (see Pelden 2012a; Deki 2012; Wangmo 2012; *The Bhutanese* 2012; BBS 2011, 2012c, 2013). For nearly three years the Drugs, Vaccines and Equipment Division (DVED 2013), the branch of the government charged with procuring authorized and accredited biomedical and traditional pharmaceuticals, had struggled to maintain supplies. A new quality and procurement protocol set out by the Drug Regulatory Authority (2012, 2013c) had restricted what could be bought and from where. This had vastly improved the quality of medicines entering Bhutan, but it had limited available products and licensed merchants. Bhutan, in comparison with some of its neighbours – China, India, Thailand and Bangladesh – was interested in comparatively small drug orders, uninspiring to foreign pharmaceutical companies that wanted bigger orders to ensure healthy profit margins.[1] The Drug Regulatory Authority's reluctance to permit cheaper medicines of dubious quality to enter Bhutan, as dictated by its legislative mandate in 'The Medicines Act' (National Assembly 2003 and MoH 2002b), further restricted their supply markets. The result was that Bhutan's selectiveness made it unattractive to pharmaceutical sellers. Petryna and Kleinman, among others, note similar issues in other countries and markets (2006: 6). They also argue for the recurring effects of such supply restrictions: 'But drug and treatment strategies also go beyond the body, affecting and potentially reshaping interpersonal, family, and community domains' (8). Such knock-on effects were occurring in Bhutan: the bottleneck of supply-frustrated doctors seeking novel ways to treat patients without their preferred tools; worried patients unable to source their prescribed medicines; and a massive headache for the Ministry of Health, which shouldered much of the blame.

What was new about the story my journalist friend was agitating to write was the alleged direct effect of these shortages on a patient, to the point of death. For the journalist, what he saw as a direct causal relationship signified a new level of culpability, and he intended to draw the nation's attention to his cousin's passing and the ministry's fatal shortcomings. He wasn't alone with his reactionary tone; even some doctors I worked with were keen for the story to break, hoping it might de-clot the supply blockages, wherever they might be. I was shown ledgers that clearly listed the drug shortages within critical medicine departments and the accompanying order forms, none of which were being filled. Pressure was building up, and this story was seen by the journalist and many hospital staff as a breaking point.

Some wanted this story to go nationwide; almost everyone wanted the problem solved. The journalist did write his story, and it was followed by other journalists, such as the article and accompanying television program from the Bhutan Broadcast Service entitled, 'Our Daughter Died because of Lack of Medicines: Parents' (2012a). The accusations rang clear. But beneath this immediate claim was a complex and multilayered patient-and-illness narrative that included a counterclaim that the medicine shortage was not to blame.[2] This contrary narrative questioned the allegation of the journalist, Neyzang's parents and many who read about the fatality in the newspapers. The Ministry of Health was quick to investigate the case thoroughly and reply to the public outcry. They couldn't conclusively say that the medicine shortage was to blame, and this was corroborated by the attending medical specialist who said that 'he [could] not really confirm that she died because of a lack of medicines as she was brought [to hospital] dead' (BBS 2013, corroborated by my own fieldnotes). As mentioned in chapter 4, the lack of autopsies in Bhutan sustains a certain ambiguity around death. Subsequently the story slowly faded from public consciousness. A family continued to grieve and the bureaucratic bottlenecking of medicines slowly worked itself out. By 2015 the issue of drug shortages neared a resolution thanks to successful negotiations between the Ministry of Health, its affiliates and international pharmaceutical suppliers, although supply chains remained vulnerable.[3]

What does this story and its active agents, both materials and persons, tell us about the changing relationships between patients, doctors, people and healing materials, specifically biomedical tools? I will delve further into this ethnographic narrative to answer this question. To understand how Neyzang's relations to materials changed due to unavoidable illness, we must first understand the biomedical concepts of her health in context with her diagnosed heart disease.

Neyzang had a heart defect. The case was serious enough and her nationalization status[4] appropriate for her to receive a fully paid referral to India in 2008. She travelled in the company of a sponsored family member and underwent a serious but successful double heart valve replacement surgery. Having recovered with the support of Indian post-surgical care, she returned to Mongar Hospital where she would receive ongoing medications as prescribed by the only medical specialist in the eastern region. Her health improved, and after a short time she became pregnant and gave birth to a healthy baby girl.

After heart valve replacement surgeries like Neyzang's, patients depend on a constant supply of medication. As a result of the lifesaving surgery, Neyzang's blood was at risk of coagulation, causing what biomedicine calls 'thrombosis', the formation of a clot inside a blood vessel that impedes flow. Heart valves that malfunction or heart chambers that receive a replacement valve are particularly susceptible to thrombosis because the surrounding tissue is particularly 'thrombogenic'. In these damaged areas the swells of blood that pause for a fraction of a second as the heart pumps have a greater potential to clot. To protect heart valve replacement patients from ventricular thrombosis, they are given anticoagulant drugs that 'interfere with the formation of blood clots. Many people refer to anticoagulants as "blood thinners"; however, [they] do not thin the blood but instead cause the blood to take longer to form a clot' (Fiumara and Goldhaber 2009: e220). The most common of these is known as Warfarin (Fiumara and Goldhaber 2009; Holbrook et al. 2005), found on the ministry's Essential Drug List (DRA 2013b). This major pharmaceutical drug is the first material subject I am placing in relation to Neyzang, the patient.

The second material is another pharmaceutical drug, known as an international normalized ratio (INR) reagent, required to monitor the levels of coagulation in the blood. Heart valve patients can't take unlimited amounts of Warfarin. They have to keep close to a set level of coagulation. Too much would restrict coagulation and risk internal bleeding (when blood can't clot); too little would cause the blood to clot in veins (Isbister et al. 2003). INR reagent tests indicate whether a patient's Warfarin levels should be raised or reduced. Without the INR reagent, doctors wouldn't know how a patient's blood was reacting to medication or how close they were to a healthy level of coagulation. There are many variants of INR reagents offered in competitive pharmaceutical markets. Some INR reagents are even offered as at-home testing kits (Sidhu and O'Kane 2001; Gardiner et al. 2005), but these are currently unavailable in Bhutan due to cost, availability and implementation feasibility.

Neyzang required both of these drugs for the healthy functioning of her heart valve replacements, so she made repeated trips to Mongar Hospital. Once a month she travelled from Khaling, four hours away by car, to test her blood with the INR reagents and get a reassessment of her Warfarin dosage. These repeated trips were also crucial because INR is sensitive to diet (Lubetsky et al. 1999). Testing and dietary advice from the medical specialist helped her to manage these risky variables. Depending on the INR reagent test results, the medical specialist would adjust her medication. She would then return home, fully understanding the importance of taking the medication according to her assigned dosage and times.

This inextricable connection to two pharmaceutical drugs and Neyzang's dependence on their availability is the first patient-material relation I want to focus on. Like many other patients in Bhutan and around the world, Neyzang relied on these materials for her survival. Shim et al. (2007, 2009) have done extensive ethnographic work with patients in similar positions of clinical dependency in North American hospitals. Their conclusions from interviews with cardiac bypass, angioplasty and stent procedure patients are helpful in comprehending the seismic shift occurring for this patient in Bhutan: 'Norms regarding what life "should be like" at particular ages are continually recalibrated to the horizon of what is clinically possible. And . . . the price of living longer entails a double-edged relationship with the clinic – it generates opportunities for bodily restoration and increased self-worth but also creates ambivalence about the value of life' (2007: 245). This latter conclusion regarding ambivalence of the value of life may not be appropriate to transplant into my ethnographic context, as Shim at al. are working with elderly patients in North American communities, a world very different from that of Neyzang and others in Bhutan. However, their conclusions are significant in other ways.

The introduction of new biomedical materials have, as Shim et al. noted, 'recalibrated . . . the horizon of what is clinically possible' (2007) for Bhutanese patients. The opportunities created by heart valve replacement surgery and the supply of complex pharmaceutical drugs have trickled down through the biomedical services to patients and their families. Horizons about what is possible and, in turn, what is expected from the biomedical services have changed drastically in the last decade as this trickling down of clinical experience has spread knowledge of biomedicine and its capabilities. This was clear in the comments made by Neyzang's father, whom I met in hospital when they arrived. He was devastated, distraught and angry. He was aware of the medication that Neyzang needed but wasn't receiving due to the drug shortages. He had tried to help his daughter by contacting hospital and private pharmacies around the eastern *dzongkhags* to locate the necessary medication, but to no avail. 'We came here before, but when we reached here there was no medicine, and another time we took a cab and came but there was still no medicine. When she did not take the medicine she would cough a lot and some blood would come out' (BBS 2012a). The Bhutan Broadcast Service reporter made the point explicit: 'The parents of the deceased blamed the hospital for not having the required drugs' (2012a). The change in horizon must also be put in temporal perspective. Shim et al.'s patients in North America have had more exposure to expanding biomedical practices throughout their lives, whereas patients in Bhutan have only in the last decade begun to understand, encounter and interpret the life-altering powers of biomedical technologies, pharmaceuticals and practices. Neyzang's father grew up in a generation that didn't have the Mongar Hospital and its advanced clinical opportunities; it was only completed in 2009. His material landscape of healing had only recently changed when his daughter visited India in 2008 and began her dependence on pharmaceuticals. Subsequently, he firmly associated the lack of healing materials with his daughter's death. This is precisely the point Shim et al. notes, that patient notions of care and quality of life are 'recalibrating' to the changes in medical materiality.

Shim et al.'s final conclusion regarding the double-edged relationship with the clinic can, with slight alterations, hold firm for the Bhutanese patients I worked with. New medical materiality and the agency they exert on patients, embodied in my example of Warfarin and the INR reagent, generate new 'opportunities for bodily restoration and increased self-worth' (2007: 245). The heart disease that afflicted Neyzang was unfortunately unavoidable. Had she been born ten years earlier, chances of referral would have been much slimmer; twenty years before and it would have been a near impossibility. As Melgaard and Dorji note, 'While patients were being sent to India since the 1940s, it was not systematic and was limited to Royal family members, court officials and senior monks only. . . . By the 1980s the number of patients being referred averaged 150 annually' (2012: 124–25). Even if, ten or twenty years ago, Neyzang had been lucky enough to get a referral, it is questionable whether the surgical technology would have been available in India or the Warfarin and INR drugs available in Mongar. Essentially her death would have been unavoidable. But new medical materiality can now offer new opportunities for bodily restoration. The double edge in this case was a challenging dependence on these materials and a contingent and continued relationship with the drugs and their supply chain. Patients such as Neyzang have very little control over either of these double edges, neither the new biomedical healing materials to which they have become accustomed nor their availability. As highlighted by the father when discussing his repeated attempts, including expensive taxi rides, to access medication, the dependence on pharmaceuticals without the ability to get them was extremely taxing on their family. This is the double edge that patients in Bhutan are facing. On the one hand new medical materials increase their chances of survival. On the other it opens up a whole new sociality of medical material dependency.

In 2012, as Mongar Hospital supplies of Warfarin and INR reagents dwindled, it wasn't just patients who felt the effects of the shortages. Doctors too had to react to the variability of supply. One medical specialist I spoke with voiced his progression of frustration and adaption. When stocks of the INR reagent ran low, he had to guess how much Warfarin to prescribe. This was risky, especially when he knew his patients might not be taking the medication at his prescribed dosages and times; variability in patient pharmaceutical behaviour was common, as many patients didn't understand the complexities and subtleties of a medication course – in comparison to biomedicine's drug consumption specificity, traditional medicine and alternative remedies could be taken in varying amounts at irregular intervals with little concern about side effects. When Warfarin stocks ran low, the doctor had to send patients home empty-handed. This had happened twice to Neyzang.

At first the doctor made every effort to access Warfarin and the INR reagent. He called many of his contacts at the ministry, the Drug, Vaccines and Equipment Division, the Drug Regulatory Authority and the Thimphu hospital. Eventually these leads ran dry, and he took the matter into his own hands. In these situations, he and a few colleagues would pile into a car and make a drug run to the border towns of the southeast, where they would shop for essential medicines in India. However, as the Drug Regulatory Authority's protocols for drug imports strengthened and their willingness to impose heavy fines and prison time increased, such activities were deemed too risky.[5] After a few years of trying hard to maintain the supply, he felt deflated and frustrated by the persisting shortages and eventually lost his will to search. He continued to prescribe Warfarin, and when his patients complained that the hospital pharmacy was out of stock, he simply told them to look elsewhere in the Mongar private pharmacies. Patients were essentially turned away from the services they had become dependent on for survival, with little hope of successfully sourcing these materials.

I want to make it very clear that I am not blaming Mongar Hospital, its staff, the Ministry of Health, the Drug Regulatory Authority, the Drug, Vaccines and Equipment Division, the Royal Government of Bhutan or any other single institution for these shortages or the death of this patient. As mentioned at the top of this section, there is not sufficient evidence to conclude that the patient's death was caused by a lack of medication. Even if it was proven, the complexity of the issues surrounding the bottleneck of supply extend way beyond a single institution and instead reach into the wider networks and the relationships between international actors, such as the many pharmaceutical companies that make and distribute these drugs. The exploration of this tragic case and the actors involved is meant to highlight the changing relationships between patients and biomedical healing materials, not to cast blame or judgement.

Arising from this narrative is an obvious yet crucial relationship between patients and materials: This patient, her doctors, and all other biomedical patients in Bhutan are now connected to international medical markets and companies, a set of relations that are likely to increase and complicate as Bhutan further develops its services.

One of the most useful works in understanding the full effect of these expanding relationships is Petryna, Lakoff and Kleinman's (2006) edited volume *Global Pharmaceuticals: Ethics, Markets, Practices*. This volume's ethnographies are 'concerned with the human consequences of pharmaceutical use and their market expansions in cross-cultural and everyday contexts', in particular the 'interests and stakes involved in the production of pharmaceuticals and their consumption in particular times and places' (Petryna and Kleinman 2006: 5). Throughout the volume, it becomes apparent that Bhutan's lack of access to international pharmaceutical markets is not an isolated case but a worrying norm for less economically developed countries. Petryna and Kleinman (2006: 6) highlight the dangers of this restricted access and its connection (or disconnection) to patient well-being and the ethics of effective and humane care in what they call a 'values gap', where

> symptoms include the growing division between populations that have access to life-saving drugs and the ability to pay for them, and populations that have neither and must rely on some other form of distribution. The gap is intensified by the choices made by industry: afflictions whose treatments are relatively easily produced and have ready markets are deemed more worthy of research and development. It is also reinforced by the subtle and not so subtle ways by which the significance of others' well-being is judged. Human experiences of suffering and its costs can have little bearing on economic measures of costs of 'morbidity' and other indicators configuring social need (Kleinman and Kleinman 1996). In other instances it is economic worth – specifically market readiness (or lack of it) – that can determine the fate of whole populations.

Bhutan's lack of 'market readiness' affected its whole population, manifested in individual patient cases. The country's inability to compete for sales attention in global pharmaceutical markets was one of the main reasons Neyzang was unable to access ready doses of Warfarin and INR reagents in Mongar. Such inequality of access in Bhutan works to highlight the argument that a 'values gap' is created between those populations that have access to medications and those that don't, as well as the end-user patients and pharmaceutical companies. This is a macro-level view of pharmaceutical ethics, operating within large international networks of pharmaceutical companies and government buyers. However, this macro-ethic erupts at the patient life-world level, most evidently in Neyzang's death, as she lacked access to the drugs she needed. As Petryna and Kleinman note, 'The gap is intensified by the choices made by industry' (2006: 6). Therefore, patients and their experiences of suffering and healing are intrinsically connected to the decisions made by these companies and the damaging results of ethical disparity between supply and need; macro-level activity and its underlying ethics affects patients at the micro level.

The effects of these connections are felt worldwide, and are often dictated in the everyday lives of patients by what Das and Das (2006: 171–205), in their contribution to the *Global Pharmaceuticals* volume, call the 'local ecologies' in which pharmaceuticals are enacted on the terms and conditions of patient and doctor socialities. Their chapter explores the issues of pharmaceutical use in a poor Delhi neighbourhood, tracing the results of the values gap as it plays out in the everyday lives of Indian patients. They use the concept of local ecologies because (202–3)

> it shows how such material processes as household cash flow, patterns of disease burden, and the availability of pharmaceuticals are integrally tied to the way that linguistic diagnostic categories come into being within specific local worlds. Within these local ecologies, everyday life is about both securing access to context and being in danger of not quite securing it. Thus, local ecologies do not produce contexts for transparency of experience but rather for the struggle over the real.

Their approach is helpful in understanding the challenges faced by the patients I worked with who were integrally tied to a growing number of biomedical pharmaceutical materials. The materials themselves gain an agency in the local ecologies or social contexts of these patients, which in turn bring other material processes into the fold of decision-making. Dialysis patients, like the one described at the beginning of this chapter, are a good case in point. The patient's survival was dependent upon a sustained relationship with a dialysis machine and the chemical dialysate. Breaking this material relationship into its component parts, the patient was reliant upon the continued supply of semipermeable membranes and the dialysate fluid that pumped out of a gallon jug, blended with his blood, and then flowed into an outlet container. Without these materials, his kidneys would break down and death would be imminent. Therefore these materials must be continually sought in international markets. The ministry must amalgamate enough funding to buy these materials. The Drug, Vaccines and Equipment Division must create a national operations unit made up of people, trucks, roads and gasoline that work together to deliver these items to the patient. These are confluences of materials, assembling in the blood flow of this patient. All these materials have agencies of their own, pushing and pulling against the other materials and the persons who want them, use them, need them.

The patient also must exert an agency of sorts to place his body in relation to these materials. In other words, this patient proactively changed his life and the socialities in which he lived. For Das and Das (2006: 203), these changing

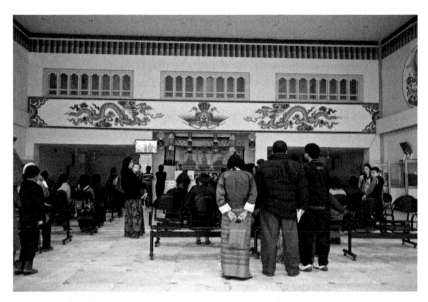

Illustration 5.2. Mongar Hospital Reception, *Mongar Hospital.* The large reception hall of Mongar Hospital.

socialities include the variables of the patient's 'local ecologies' that 'produce contexts for the struggle over the real'. The dialysis patient moved from Trashigang, four hours away, to take up accommodation next to the hospital. He was required to put his body into the bed next to the dialysis machine and filtrate his blood through its tubes three times a week. He gave up farming, his income, regular family contact, his connections to familiar landscapes, and sacred geographies filled with village deities and spirits to be close to this machine. He could no longer leave Mongar for long periods of time without risking kidney failure. He was lucky to receive hospital patient accommodation, a simple apartment made specifically for patients who must upheave their worlds to chase survival. Many patients will not receive this gift from the government and will have to work out regular transport or local accommodation. This patient changed his entire social world to sustain a new relationship with this machine; his 'local ecology' was changed forever.

Both the heart valve and dialysis narratives are examples of patients changing their behaviours in the face of new biomedical technology and of the relationships formed between the body and its curative functions. Other patients regularly do the same thing, but in less spectacular ways. Many take prescription medicines, made available in hospital and street-side pharmacies. There has also been the influx of nutriceuticals, drugs that tread a fine line between pharmaceuticals and natural products, much to the annoyance of the Drug Regulatory Authority, which wants greater transparency in medical categorization. Emerging medical materials and associated practices are changing lives. Recalling Shim et al. (2007), this is a changing horizon of healthcare, where new clinical solutions are enacted, understood and engaged by patients. These technologies are relatively new. The changes to behaviour are accelerating as knowledge and practice of new biomedical materiality ramp up and secure a foothold in the healing narratives and healthcare-seeking behaviours of patients nationwide. The increased use of biomedicine is saving more lives in Bhutan and reducing suffering. Melgaard and Dorji (2012), in their history of the improvements of national health statistics like morbidity, child mortality and other health indicators (2012: 72–79), offer ample evidence of this. The increase in the number of surgeries in Bhutan can also be investigated; likewise the myriad of materials, environments, specialization and training required to perform such medical procedures. Little to nothing is known about how Bhutanese patients understand these new services. With the dramatic expansion of patients' use of these growing services, more socio-cultural research is warranted into how the changing relations affect patients.

Conclusion: Practical Applications for Medical Materiality

This chapter has looked at the changing effects of biomedical materiality on patients, specifically in instances when medicine dependence changed patient's lives. The narration of Neyzang who tragically died due to complications with a heart valve replacement she received in 2008 provided evidence to this. The issues of accessibility were teased out through the immersive context of a pharmaceutical drug shortage that was underway during my fieldwork. Although it remains inconclusive whether the Neyzang died due to the drug shortage, her narrative served to explore how she, her family and the doctors that treated her were inextricably connected to international pharmaceutical markets and the economic, political and social powers that negotiated and arranged these relations. The effects of these relations were laid bare when the medicines were taken away. Parents and family members voiced their anger at the Ministry of Health for not providing the services they were promised. The ministry and Drug Regulatory Authority strengthened their efforts and claims to provide safe pharmaceuticals rather than flooding hospitals with unaccredited medications. Doctors implemented drastic plans to increase the availability of medications but came up against sustainability issues due to regulation. It became evident through these actions and responses that biomedical pharmaceuticals and access to them had become an ingrained and important materiality for patients, carers and the government, with new expectations of supply being harboured and supported by all parties. While new health material access meant patients such as Neyzang had a fighting chance at life, it came with the double-edged dependence on pharmaceuticals and therefore on the tenuous supply of these materials and the macro-ethics that guided the pharmaceutical suppliers.

If biomedical materiality plays a key role in patient healthcare-seeking behaviour, how might this information help Bhutan's healthcare services? Recalling chapter 3's discussion of parents oscillating between bringing their children into hospital or keeping them at home for alternative healing rituals, the allure of the hospital is in its materiality, a collective perception of curative technology, complementary to the religious rituals. In those examples, wavering between effective and appropriate materials of healing caused healthcare-seeking delays that were bemoaned by hospital doctors, resulting in debates regarding 'appropriate care'.

Patients' perception of materials and their efficacy are central to how and when they seek certain forms of healthcare. Patient perception and resulting motivations are areas in which the Ministry of Health and other healthcare institutions in Bhutan could engage practically in order to encourage patients to visit. My finding rings clear: patients are attracted to efficacious-looking healthcare materiality. In other words, patients are drawn to things that they think will work. Therefore, more advertising that highlights effective materials for healthcare in the health centres and public health announcements of Bhutan could prompt patients to visit clinics in a timely manner and find appropriate care.

Discussing practical applications of materiality to the healthcare institutions of Bhutan brings up two important points. The first is that such biomedical and traditional materiality, on some level, is juxtaposed with alternative practices and their materials, such as the blades used in cutting and sucking (chapters 1 and 4) or the strings placed on pregnant women's bellies as described in this chapter. Materials ascribed to different service types of healthcare are often pitted against each other, with proponents of each making a series of arguments for and against their use and promotion. The curative techniques deployed by *ja né* healers are a good case in point. As argued in chapter 4, alternative practices play a meaningful and agentive role in patients' experiences of healing, so it would be wise for any promotion of materiality in juxtaposition with these alternatives to be sensitive to the value placed on these alternatives by patients and communities. Any promotion of biomedical or traditional materiality should be mindful of the other types of materials patients engage with daily.

The second point is a caveat that comes from the many studies in medical anthropology of the detrimental effects of medical advertising around the world. Mol (2008) has taken a focused look at how advertising for diabetes treatments can guide patients into a marketplace of proliferating choice rather than effective care. David Healy (2006) has shown how motives based on financial considerations for such advertising have often been to blame for ethical breaches between pharmaceutical companies and their customers; he gives as his pertinent example the marketing of anti-depressants in the United States in the 1980s and 1990s. There is a vast library of such studies, with a clear warning: large, centralized and well-funded advertising doesn't always have the patient's best interest at heart. Any direct marketing of medical materials to patients by Bhutan's health institutions will have to be transparent and accountable.

That said, promotion of and education in appropriate medical materiality to their patients could be a productive approach by all healthcare institutions. Patients could benefit from sensitive education enabling responsible healthcare-seeking behaviour and consequent betterment of patient healthcare experiences. The increase, diversification and complication of medical materiality in Bhutan is likely set to continue, with the Ministry of Health improving services and technology on a daily basis. I would argue that a population properly knowledgeable about new materials is likely to display a more appropriate, effective and timely response to illness.

Notes

1. To combat the lack of seller interest in the Bhutanese market, the Drug Regulatory Authority actively tried to market itself as a 'charity' case, highlighting the country's poverty status. It was thought that if competitive capital markets wouldn't sell to Bhutan, then perhaps they could target a more 'humanitarian' market. Bhutan does not have a history of placing itself in such charity-donor relations, preferring a more independent and self-assured stance. The charity tactic deployed by the Drug Regulatory Authority and the Ministry of Health thus demonstrates the severity of the drug shortage issue and how the political actors were willing to change policies to solve it.
2. I make a side note here to the vast and valuable work done by a host of medical anthropologists on the topic of medical access inequality due to variability in income and prosperity levels. Work such as Chen et al. (1993), Desjarlais et al. (1995), Kim et al. (2000) and Farmer (2001, 2004) have demonstrated how inequities of health and access to healthcare build on socio-economic, cultural and political divisions, often between countries, income groups and ethnic minorities. Bhutan fits into this literature. For example, wealthy persons in Thimphu have greater access to foreign referrals, if not through the official system that works hard to maintain equality in case-priority referrals, then through the leveraging of personal funds for medical tourism to places like India or Bangkok. The history of royal family members and elites having access to national and foreign medical care is well known (McKay 2007; Melgaard and Dorji 2012). However, in the case discussed here, I would argue that while poverty levels do play a role in the challenges of accessing medication – for example, the inability to travel to India regularly to buy them – this particular patient was on a relatively equal par with the rest of the population who relied on the Ministry of Health and its clinical services to deliver medications. If this patient couldn't access drugs, neither could many others all around Bhutan due to Drug, Vaccines and Equipment Division shortages.
3. See MoH 2013: 11–12 for the ministry's report on how the drug shortage problem was resolved.
4. See chapter 2 for an explanation of the national identity requirements for patient referrals abroad.
5. Cross-border transit of other materials has also become a growing concern for the Royal Government of Bhutan, with the restriction of tobacco, alcohol and drugs taking centre stage. For example, in 2011, a monk was jailed for three years for smuggling cigarettes into Bhutan (Buncombe and Waraich 2011; Pem 2011).

Conclusion
Assembling Patient Multiples and Complementary Logics of Care

Deconstructing Rigid Practices for Flexible Patients

From the outset of this ethnographic exploration into Bhutanese healing narratives, I foregrounded patient-practice relations in three assemblages of healthcare: biomedical, traditional and alternative. I identified these three categories in the course of following patients who sought amelioration of health-related sufferings from their different diagnostic, treatment and material solutions. Not only did patients draw attention to differences between these three types of practices – navigating and engaging them in different ways – but the supporting political, economic, ethical and social networks were also structured along these lines of division. This was never clearer than in the differences between institutionalization (biomedical and traditional) and non-institutionalization (alternative). These differences of institutionalization went on to affect resource distribution, legislation, accreditation, access, media coverage and national health policies for each of these practice sets. These three categories of practice were real for the patients who used them and were distinguishable in the ways they were approached and managed within healthcare-seeking narratives. Relationships with the three practices would also result in different treatment and amelioration outcomes for patients, rendering again a difference, this time through direct experience and practice interaction.

While these assemblages of healthcare have in some ways defined the parameters of the patient narratives explored here, it's important to recognize the mutability and permeability of these categories. I have purposely avoided calling these practices 'systems' of any kind. To do so would call upon too deliberate and rigid a structure that ignores the variations within and between the practices, as well as the ways that patients enact and experience them. This is an issue well addressed in medical anthropology's literature and history.

Medical anthropology's exploration of pluralism between medical systems was groundbreaking in the 1970s, with Charles Leslie's *Asian Medical Systems: A Comparative Study* (1976) and its complementing theoretical publication (1978) creating discursive space for the coexistence of healing regimes, specifically biomedicine and traditional Chinese medicine in China and Ayurvedic medicine and Unami medicine in India. For the first time anthropologists started to engage with system plurality in healthcare, in non-Western societies (Janzen 1982; Ohnuki-Tierney 1984; Selin 2003; Stoner 1986; Crandon-Malamud 1993), in the West (Baer 2001, 1987; Sharma 1992; Cant and Sharma 1996) and on a global scale (Baer et al. 2003; Coreil and Mull 1990; Nichter and Nichter 1996; Strathern and Stewart 2010). But critiques of system theory in line with postmodern thinking soon questioned the notion of isolated modalities of practice that fit neatly into system categorizations. For example, Press (1980), in his work *De-emphasizing the Exotic in the Clinic: Strategies for Enhancing the Utility of Clinical Anthropology*, showed how medical systems had different meanings in different studies (Johannessen 2006: 3), concluding that the overall idea of medical pluralism was flawed due to its reliance on systems that were more open and adaptable than were described.

Later ethnographic work departed from focuses on systems and chose instead the body and self, and their relationships, as subjects of exploration. Scheper-Hughes and Lock (1987), among others, defined the trajectory for such body–self interfaces by outlining three analytical angles of research: the 'social body' (as constituted by socialities), the 'individual body' (that of phenomenological perception and conception, e.g., Csordas 1997a, 1997b and 2002) and the 'body politic' (as organized by social, political and economic regulations). Many works, too numerous and off-topic to go into here, continued this line of analytical thought and ethnographic focus, preferring to look at the types of bodies created by practices rather than the conglomerations of the practices themselves, or what Leslie would have called 'medical systems'.

In recognition of these theoretical trajectories, as well as the mass amount of complementary material produced by many other medical anthropologists, I have steered clear of categorizing healing practices as 'systems'. I have also moved away from centring this ethnography on the practices themselves given the issues of limiting subjects like 'practice' and 'medical knowledge' to singular interpretations or occurrences, given that the literature has shown that multiplicity and flux of such subjects is the norm.

Instead, I have focused on the patient-subject. More specifically, this book has aimed to learn how Bhutanese patients are affected by the contexts of healthcare that frame their diagnosis, treatment and illness understandings. Rather than using the body as the locus of study, I selected the social category of 'patient' by following Mol's (2003) theory of 'enactment', which looks at how subjects emerge or are created by the 'doing' of practice. But enactment is not limited to patient–practice relations alone; it incorporates the body-theories noted earlier. I also looked at the ways that patients enact different notions of health, which are then affiliated to different modalities of care. Also, folding in the insights of the 'social body', I included the enactment of bodies within different socialities of health and practice. The enactment of practices, healths and bodies ultimately defines what I came to understand as a 'patient' in Bhutan.

The first chapter set out this analytical imperative in attempting to define what a patient was in the Bhutanese context. It began, as many other works on patient healthcare-seeking narratives do, with the observation that patients in Bhutan were using a vast array of healing practices to respond to illness. In doing so, they were placing themselves in relation to differing sets of medical and healing knowledge and practice. These relations and the everyday treatment and consultation activities that followed constituted enactments of these practices, affecting people's phenomenologies, body-knowledges and ethics, thus forming conceptions of 'patient-hood'.

These analytical conclusions were evidenced by Pema's healthcare-seeking narrative as she underwent surgery in the biomedical hospital for nasal pain before moving on to the traditional medicine hospital for follow-up treatments. Her deliberate switch between the biomedical and traditional services was not only emblematic of practice-plurality offered in the two-option state healthcare services but also of how patients can have multifarious conceptions of health and aetiologies of disease; in switching hospitals, Pema also spoke about how her illness had multiple 'sides' to it, one of which could not be treated by one of the hospitals, requiring attention from the other. Although the symptoms remained the same, she described having multiple healths, each of which required specific attention and care. She then complicated this multiple health concept by revealing a third illness caused by poisoning, requiring a practice known as 'cutting and sucking' from an alternative healer. This third tangent of practice unfurled another side of her health, this time affecting a different body than her previous illness. She bisected her body, both conceptually and phenomenologically.

The complexity of this narrative that echoed those of other patients I worked with in Bhutan and Pema's enactment of practice, health and body multiples led me to conclude that Pema was a 'patient multiple'. She was multiples of a patient-subject at once, sometimes overlapping and commensurable, at other times distinct and incommensurable. Finally, I argued that this patient multiplicity was kept cohesive due to its agentive meaningfulness in the healthcare-seeking decision-making process and subsequent narratives of Pema and other patients. Enacting multiples of patient-hood through practices, healths and bodies provided meaning to illness itself, as well as the challenging task of seeking amelioration. Patient multiplicity is an active lens on illness experiences, through which patients can view themselves and their desires for healthiness. It is this agentive meaningfulness that keeps patients coherent in the face of ethical, institutional and knowledge differences between practices, conceptions of health and bodies.

Having formulated a conceptualization of a patient that works within the context of Bhutan, chapter 2 explored the effects of traditional medicine, the state-run institutionalized and nationalized complementary services, on sick persons. The National Traditional Medicine Hospital and its nationwide units have rapidly expanded their service locations, traditional medicines and human resources to meet a growing demand among the Bhutanese population. With help of preliminary quantitative studies such as Lhamo (2011, 2010) and Lhamo and Nebel (2011), it is possible to conclude that most people in Bhutan know of and have used these traditional services. Lhamo's findings show that '82% of the people in general said that they have heard about sowa rigpa', especially those in urban settings (90 percent) against rural dwellers (74 percent) (2011: 17). Given that only 10 percent of the population still has no access to primary health services (NSB 2012: 2) the knowledge of traditional medicine as an accessible service in the national population is relatively high. I argued that this was achieved through the standardization, nationalization and professionalization of traditional services at the state level, which created a national hierarchic network of care that patients were learning to use in response to illness. A commitment to 'medical integration' of a two-option healthcare service in the early 1960s, when the Ministry of Health was founded, sustained funding and policy support for this nationalization process.

While patient multiplicity is very much enacted from the part of the patient, there are agents of healthcare, specifically the institutionalized biomedical and traditional state services, that aim to territorialize the discursive space defining what a patient 'officially' is. Much work has been done on biomedical and biological citizenship, categories of state identity created through biomedical science, often deployed to legitimize access to services or create a body-politic tied with national agendas. Petryna (2002) was one example used here to demonstrate the power such biological citizenship plays in patients' lives, as it does in Bhutan: the international referral system for treatment in India was a case in point. I argued that the institution of traditional medicine is also producing what I coined a 'bio-traditional citizenship', whereby patients are defined through a *sowa rigpa* knowledge infused with Bhutanese state identity. The computerization of patient records and subsequent use in reporting of national healthcare statistics, the growing ability of patients to navigate the national clinic network and the ethics surrounding disease codification and diagnosis are all efforts towards a bio-traditional citizenship.

The results of these efforts are twofold. First, they are sustaining and expanding a healthcare service complementary to the biomedical services. Without state support and patient participation in their own bio-traditional citizenship, such services would remain sidelined and underdeveloped. Instead, carving out a citizenship identity specific to *sowa rigpa* is helping the services gain traction in healthcare ethics, policy and, most importantly, a patient population that is growing hungrier and more demanding of its state services. Therefore bio-traditional citizenship is helping to cement traditional medicine in the state offerings of a two-option medical service. Second, it flexes and exercises the patient multiple. When arriving at a hospital and deciding between biomedical or traditional services, patients are inadvertently participating in a multiplication process. They are sliding between knowledges and practices and in doing so furthering their ability to be multiple subjects in a practice-plural context.

Given the evidence that state services are growing, this is a process and skill that patients are likely to get better at and will require in the future if they are to make appropriate decisions about which practice they are going to use and when.

The third chapter picked up the latter point of 'appropriate decision-making' by looking at the effect of practice-plurality on patients as they attempted to decide which treatments to use. Patients in Bhutan, especially in rural areas where accessibility to institutionalized services is challenging due to transport, time, topographic and cost barriers, often engage in complex decision-making processes about when, how and where to treat illness. I explored these processes by focusing on two ethnographic narratives revolving around Mongar and its Eastern Regional Referral Hospital.

The first involved a new mother and father, Tshomo and Sonam respectively, who gave birth to their first child in their small village BHU. Unfortunately the mother's milk took a few days to come in, and because the parents did not receive adequate guidance from their community or healthcare centre, the baby became critically dehydrated and jaundiced. The lack of support was compounded by two factors: First the parents were relatively isolated from the community because they were teachers placed in a remote and unfamiliar social setting and thus disconnected and unfamiliar with their neighbours – an issue that many civil-service employees stationed in unfamiliar locations all over Bhutan experience. Second, they were teachers, well educated and practiced in public health knowledge. This false confidence was met by a practical unfamiliarity with breastfeeding and neonatal care. The result was a slow deliberation over whether or not to visit hospital, as well as over when to introduce the village *lama* and his *rim dro* practices to the treatment process. Eventually the parents decided to go to hospital at the behest of the mother's sister, and the baby recovered in the intensive care unit. At the same time a *rim dro* was held in their home to complement the hospital treatment.

The second narrative follows the story of Dechen, a three-year-old girl who suffered from what is described in biomedical terms as osteomyelitis in her left arm, caused from what the parents identified as an angered *yül lha* (village or territorial deity). The parents kept Dechen home over four months as the pain worsened, conducting a series of *rim dro* that attempted to appease the *yül lha*. By the fourth month Dechen was severely ill, transposing the sickness into a greater state of 'acuteness', as perceived by the parents. They decided to take her to Mongar Hospital where, due to the complicated and recurring nature of a disease like osteomyelitis, she required multiple operations and month-long stays. Meanwhile, the parents continued conducting *rim dro* at home, maintaining the logic of the disease's spiritual aetiology. In having to return to hospital many times and continuing *rim dro* at home, they sustained a spiritually conceived logic of care melded with biomedical curative technologies.

Both of these narratives could be dissected and analyzed in numerous ways. I chose to focus on what these narratives reveal about decision-making processes and an emerging ethics of 'appropriate care', a topical question in contemporary public health programming in Bhutan. I argued that the Ministry of Health was attempting to territorialize the discursive space for what is 'appropriate healthcare-seeking behaviour'. Biomedical and traditional doctors want patients to come to them first before taking another type of treatment, if any at all. Conversely, alternative healers and their supporters continue to encourage the use of their practices, and they recommend that patients visit hospital in conjunction with their treatment. These pushes and pulls are exerted on patients as they were on the parents in my two narratives. I concluded that patient use of multiple practices is an important part of meaningful healthcare-seeking behaviour for the Bhutanese, and allowing them to participate in patient multiplicity again provides agency in the decision-making process and in experiences of illness and amelioration. But this raises the question of how to ensure that the positives from practice choice are not eroded by other health-damaging aspects, such as the near death of the baby after delay.

To answer this question I reiterated Mol's (2008) call for a 'logic of care' over a 'logic of choice'. All healthcare providers, biomedical, traditional, and alternative, would need to focus their efforts on providing healthcare solutions that emphasize effective and timely care and not just diversify the treatment options available. However, given the importance of patient multiplicity, this does not mean simply elevating one practice above all others. It is more about arranging practice-plurality in such a way to ensure that patients move fluidly between treatments, gaining the health and mental benefits of this multiplicity without restricting access to vital care. This is a challenging endeavour given the imperative of saving and improving lives, which is at the top of the agenda for the Ministry of Health and its collaborators. However, the patient narratives provided in this ethnography show peoples' ability to cohesively use practice, health and body multiplicity to respond to illnesses. Reorienting healthcare practices around patients and their particular wants and values may then provide a more effective service provision, incorporating the agency and power of patients themselves. In the case of healthcare-seeking behaviour, it becomes more a question of treatment arrangement rather than one or the other.

Chapter 4 expanded the ethnographic inquiry into healthcare decision-making in Mongar and its surrounding villages by examining the effects of alternative practices on patients. This chapter began at a wider national perspective, tracing the discourses surrounding the activities of alternative healers and some of the contemporary attitudes and pressures guiding their work and, in turn, how patients were engaging their practices. It then zoomed in on a particular type of disease known as *ja né*, which has three different iterations. The first is defined by traditional medicine and the *sowa rigpa* canon. This disease is affiliated with changing environments or behaviours, often attributed to travel to southern areas such as India where cholera, dysentery or malaria can be more easily picked up. The second form of *ja né* is used by the Dzongkha Development Commission, the Royal Government of Bhutan, the Ministry of

Health and its biomedical public health programmes to describe avian flu. For Ugyen, a young student who learnt about public health through government schooling and television, this was the predominant interpretation of *ja né*. The third form of the disease is more of a catchall category, with many different versions or symptom explainers. It describes illnesses relating to the groin, genitals and midsection of the body, presenting symptoms similar to what biomedicine would call urinary tract infections or sexually transmitted diseases. However, I made the important point that while this is an apt and arguably accurate interpretation of this *ja né* in biomedical terms, it would be presumptuous and ethnographically erroneous to compress and translate this disease as such. Instead, *ja né* has its own linguistic, social and healing space amongst patients and healers that has nothing to do with biomedical interpretations. It is this distinctive disease that requires the skills of *ja né* healers.

The final section of this chapter explored the practice of removing this third form of *ja né* by the sucking of genital discharge from both male and female patients, as performed by one Mongar healer. It discussed how this was performed orally, exposing both healer and patient to a series of risks, including *dug* (poisoning), sexual assault, charges of sexual assault and cross-infection. This practice was then framed again in a national perspective with media, patients and pundits sharing opinions on the practice, with many reacting negatively to a case of sexual assault by a healer on a young female patient. The pressures and controversies of such a practice were explored in the context of such national attention; however, differing opinions and patients' continued use of *ja né* healers, even once controversially in the intensive care unit of Mongar Hospital, demonstrate a strong demand for such healers and underline their important role in the healthcare-seeking narratives of some Bhutanese patients. I concluded that in the face of such polarizing opinions, the use of *ja né* healers by patients who navigate these controversies and the differing opinions of what *ja né* is and how it has to be treated exemplify the enactment of patient multiplicity and again the competency of patients to cohesively manage multiplicity amongst disparate healthcare opinions.

The fifth chapter added the important analytical and ethnographic perspective of healing materials and their effect on patients. While other chapters focused mainly on practice–patient relations, this one looked at how the materials deployed in different healing scenarios would go on to create, sustain and change patients in modern day Bhutan. It argued that these changing material landscapes constitute agentive non-human actors in processes of patient-enactment and decision-making.

This argument was explored through a disturbing patient narrative, that of Neyzang, a female patient who died in the context of a national drug shortage. After undergoing a double heart valve replacement surgery, she was dependent on anticoagulant drugs, which were lacking in supply in Mongar Hospital. Although her death cannot be conclusively linked to the lack of drugs, the complaints and narratives expounded by family, carers and media around this tragedy elucidate the changing roles of materials in patients' lives. First this story emphasized the new medical horizons to which patients are becoming accustomed. New forms of medical materials and technologies are changing the life and care narratives of patients and their families. Second, new dependencies on these materials pose new risks and emerging ethics, as revealed when the materials, in this case anticoagulant pharmaceuticals, were unavailable due to supply constraints that spanned local, national and global scales. Following Shim et al. (2007, 2009) I argued that while new biomedical materials are creating new horizons for what is clinically possible and aiding in giving new hope to patients, the healthcare infrastructure in Bhutan makes consistent supply challenging and thus situations of dependence precarious. The increase of pharmaceutical dependency, for example in the case of the dialysis patient, is causing new ethical and practical conundrums for patients and healthcare services. Either patients have to change their entire lives to get closer to these materials, as with the dialysis patient, or they have to hope that access can be maintained in rural, hard-to-reach communities, as in the case with Neyzang. Ultimately new biomedical materiality affects patients' experiences of illness and healing in offering hope, but with an undercurrent of unreliability, and also changes how they structure their entire lives around such relations.

The five chapters are held together by the common themes of patient emergence and healthcare decision-making behaviour. In placing a well-defined notion of a patient (chapter 1) in the foreground of institutionalized traditional practices (chapter 2), decision-making (chapter 3), alternative practices (chapter 4) and medical materials (chapter 5), I attempted to offer an well-rounded description of what it means to be a patient in Bhutan and how relations to these relatively new aspects of their healing narratives go on to affect their experience of suffering and healing. The next section outlines some conclusions drawn from the exploration of these narratives.

Patient Multiplicity in a Logic of Care

I made an assertion in chapter 1 that has become a conclusion of this book, that patient subjectivities in Bhutan constitute a type of 'patient multiple'. This is a conceptualization of a person where the enactment of multiple practices, conceptions of health and bodies, spanning across illnesses, symptoms, curative activities and healing, require sick persons to be multiple patients in relation to the diverse knowledge and practices they engage with. Additionally, people are capable of enacting patient multiplicities simultaneously and without much contestation between opposing subjectivities or conceptions of health. In most cases, patients were very capable of remaining coherent in the face of subject-multiplicity. Even more so, they would find agentive meaningfulness in expressing or experiencing their illness through multiple patient subjectivities, encouraging a more inclusive and personal participation in suffering and healing.

It's tempting from this conclusion to assume that Bhutanese patients manage their healthcare, experiences of suffering and healing, and their conceptions of health in a 'holistic' fashion. The practice-plural world in which these patients live may also hint that patients have 'holistic' treatment options in which all sides of their physical, spiritual and mental well-being are cared for. However, I would strongly oppose this conceptualization of both patient subjectivity and the ethnographic context of healthcare practices in Bhutan. While patient multiplicity and practice-plurality do diversify the practices, healths and bodies engaged by patients, this does not necessarily satisfy all the needs or wants of a human being. The term 'holistic' implies that all parts of a patient-whole are tended to. This is not the case in Bhutan, where many instances of practice fail to ameliorate illness, leaving the patient feeling unattended to. The most striking example of this was the death of the Haa patient mentioned in chapter 3, who was failed by the lack of an effective institutional referral system. While she had access to biomedical, traditional and alternative practices, she still perished. This demonstrates that a patient multiplicity that hints at a holistic healthcare context may be just as dangerous or damaging in certain instances as a one-track healing option. What comes out of practice-plurality is the challenging scenario of decision-making, as seen in chapter 3 and the case in Haa. Therefore I would urge readers of this ethnography not to imagine patients as fully cared for within my arguments of patient multiplicity but to rather place such subjects in the complicated and challenging situations of healthcare-seeking and decision-making in which they live, suffer, heal and die.

This leads me to my main conclusion. Patients' experiences of healing are created not only by the practices they use, by the health conceptions they call upon to understand their illnesses or by which bodies emerge but also by the ways that they manage, layer, sort, order and relate their patient multiplicity. In the case of Tshomo and Sonam, the parents from chapter 3 who were considering visiting Mongar Hospital for their dehydrated newborn child and conducting a religious ceremony, there was not a choice between practices; they considered both to be potentially effective in treating their child. It was more a case of arranging and managing these therapeutic options as well as the biomedical and spiritual knowledges that informed them. They were most likely going to use the hospital and the religious rituals. Less a matter of one or the other, it was more a combination of both, into an actionable response.

Another way of viewing this is to see Tshomo and Sonam navigating and organizing patient multiplicity into a decisive set of actions. As different patient multiples emerge, they are not chosen one from another but rather assembled and then acted upon. The slow response of these parents and the mass complaint from doctors about patients' tardy presentation reflects that the process of assemblage of the patient multiple takes time, effort and consideration, and even more so when the illness is chronic rather than acute. The same can be said for alternative practices; I recall my finding that alternative healers also complained that patients came too late, again highlighting the role of patient multiplicity management in the realm of alternative practices as well. Additionally, over time and through the course of illnesses, the patient multiple can be reassembled or reshuffled, as in the case of Pema in chapter 1 who changed her view of the aetiology of her nasal condition. Processes of assembling are not momentary or static, but rather constant, reoccurring and compounding. I conclude that patient healthcare-seeking and decision-making behaviour is a process of assembling, navigating and managing patient multiplicity rather than decision-making between practices and knowledges.

How can this conclusion be applied in terms of helping Bhutanese patients and their carers better understand patients and deliver effective healthcare services? To answer this I would call upon Mol's (2008) critique of healthcare structures that value a 'logic of choice' over a 'logic of care'. In her final chapter she explores what it means to be a patient, or as she calls 'an actor', in both logics (2008: 85).

> In the logic of choice an actor is someone who makes decisions. In order to make decisions actors have to consider the relevant arguments and weigh up the advantages and disadvantages of the options available. This is not easy and all but impossible if you have a fever, are in coma, or if you are shaking with fear.

This ethnography has shown many examples of these decision-making processes for patients and how difficult the decisions can be. From the practice-plural context of Bhutan has emerged an ethical discourse concerning what are and are not 'appropriate decisions'. These become problems when healthcare providers frame in a logic of choice the services they provide and set the patient healthcare-seeking narrative in that frame as well. Practices and decisions are set against each other, with little consideration of how they may be practically complementary. Furthermore, issues of incommensurability dominate the arguments for practice integration. But as this book explored at the outset, patients don't necessarily divide practices as neatly as service providers do, who are concerned with this logic of choice. Healthcare literature as discussed in the introduction demonstrated these juxtaposed and delineated practice divisions. What I called 'patient cross-over' between practices was rather the norm for patients. This fits into the idea of patient multiplicity, where sick persons are managing and assembling their differing practices, healths and bodies into an effective response. These are practical modes of dealing with illness, resembling what Mol would call their logic of care (2008: 86):

> In the logic of care being an actor is primarily a practical matter. This does not mean that nobody ever needs to make choices. Instead, in this logic 'making a choice' appears as yet another practical task.

As patients manage their multiplicity, assembling them into practical responses to illness, they may cross over many healthcare knowledges and practices, disregarding the ethical, scientific or political incommensurability between them.

Their concern is to get effective care, not to choose this or that practice. Therefore, the patient multiple as an assembling process is in itself a logic of care, as Mol puts it, 'a practical matter' (2008: 86).

If patients are multiple, and if in managing this multiplicity they use more a logic of care than of choice, then healthcare practices that align themselves with these logics of care will more likely approach patients on their own terms and potentially make effective use of how the patient conceives of their own healing and suffering. Focusing on a logic of care will also aid patients in making decisions about which practice to use and when. Rather than drawing lines between practices, something patients are not inclined to do, they will ask themselves what will provide the best care for how they are ailing. Practices that then present the most attractive 'care' options will undoubtedly attract more patients.

I made this point in a slightly different way at the end of chapter 5, calling for the biomedical and traditional institutional practices to rethink the way they attract patients to their doors, sensitively and wisely using the allure of medical materials. My vague use of the terms 'sensitive and wise' can now get specific. If the Ministry of Health were to advertise materials to attract patients, they would have to do so from a logic of care, not of choice. These materials should demonstrate how the institutions can provide care, rather than pitting new materials against old ones, or perhaps against alternative practices. While presenting material choice to patients might at first be attractive, like having a hundred cereals to choose from at a supermarket, such diversification of choice can be disruptive to providing and promoting effective care. Given that the process of assembling the patient multiple is about a logic of care, materials that fit into this logic are more likely to draw patients' attention.

A logic of care will also open space for practices to work in complement to, rather than in competition against, one another. This leads to a greater possibility of integration between biomedical and traditional practices, as well as valuing and constructively incorporating alternative practices. By focusing on patient multiplicity, healthcare providers can remain open to the utility of other forms of care as well as their own, and they can constructively integrate these perspectives and practices into their treatment of patients.

By aligning themselves to the patient perspective, one of multiplicity, Bhutan's healthcare providers, both institutional and non-institutional, might better tailor their care to incorporate the ways that contemporary Bhutanese patients understand their own health and healing experiences. To do so would not only improve their quality of life and effectuate healing but also support patients as they grapple with challenging and complex decision-making processes. Ultimately a logic of care complements the assembly and management of patient multiplicity, increasing patient capacity for effective healthcare decision-making.

Bibliography

Adams, Vincanne. 2001. 'The Sacred in the Scientific: Ambiguous Practices of Science in Tibetan Medicine.' *Cultural Anthropology* 16(4) (November): 542–75.

——. 2002a. 'Establishing Proof: Translating "Science" and the State in Tibetan Medicine.' In *New Horizons in Medical Anthropology: Essays in Honour of Charles Leslie*, ed. Charles M. Leslie, Mark Nichter and Margaret M. Lock, 200–220. Oxon: Psychology Press.

——. 2002b. 'Randomized Controlled Crime Postcolonial Sciences in Alternative Medicine Research.' *Social Studies of Science* 32(5–6) (1 December): 659–90. doi:10.1177/030631270203200503.

Adams, Vincanne, Suellen Miller, Sienna Craig, Arlene Samen, Nyima, Sonam, Droyoung, Lhakpen and Michael Varner. 2005. 'The Challenge of Cross-Cultural Clinical Trials Research: Case Report from the Tibetan Autonomous Region, People's Republic of China.' *Medical Anthropology Quarterly* 19(3) (September): 267–89.

Adams, Vincanne, Suellen Miller, Sienna Craig, Sonam, Nyima, Droyoung, Phuoc V. Le and Micheal Varner. 2007. 'Informed Consent in Cross-Cultural Perspective: Clinical Research in the Tibetan Autonomous Region, PRC.' *Culture, Medicine and Psychiatry* 31(4) (December): 445–72. doi:10.1007/s11013-007-9070-2.

Adams, Vincanne, Mona Schrempf and Sienna R. Craig (eds.). 2010. *Medicine between Science and Religion: Explorations on Tibetan Grounds.* New York: Berghahn Books.

Al Jazeera. 2010. 'Interview with Prime Minister Jigme Thinley, Bhutan.' Web video. 101 East – Bhutan's Prime Minister. AlJazeera.net. http://english.aljazeera.net/video/.

Allen, Julie. 2012. *The Unicode Standard Version 6.1: Core Specification.* Mountain View, CA: Unicode Consortium.

Allison, Elizabeth. 2004. 'Spiritually Motivated Natural Resources Protection in Eastern Bhutan.' In *The Spider and the Piglet: Proceedings of the First International Seminar on Bhutan Studies*, ed. Karma Ura and Sonam Kinga, 529–63. Thimphu: Centre for Bhutan Studies.

Ardussi, John. 1999. 'The Rapprochement between Bhutan and Tibet under the Enlightened Rule of Sde-srid XIII Shes-rab-dbang-phyug (R.1744-63).' *Journal of Bhutan Studies* 1 (Autumn). http://www.bhutanstudies.org.bt/publications/journal-of-bhutan-studies/.

——. 2000. 'Formation of the State of Bhutan ('Brug Gzhung) in the 17th Century and Its Tibetan Antecedents.' *The Relationship between Religion and State in Traditional Tibet Conference.* Lumbini, Nepal.

Ardussi, John. 2004. 'Formation of the State of Bhutan ('Brug Gzhung) in the 17th Century and Its Tibetan Antecedents.' *Journal of Bhutan Studies* 11: 10–32.
———. 2008. 'Gyalse Tenzin Rabgye and the Celebration of Tshechu in Bhutan.' In *Written Treasures of Bhutan: Mirror of the Past and Bridge to the Future; Proceedings of the First International Conference on the Rich Scriptural Heritage of Bhutan*, ed. John Ardussi and Sonam Tobgay, 1–24. Thimphu: National Library of Bhutan.
Ardussi, John, and Françoise Pommaret (eds.). 2007. *Bhutan: Traditions and Changes; PIATS 2003: Tibetan Studies: Proceedings of the Tenth Seminar of the International Association for Tibetan Studies, Oxford, 2003.* Brill's Tibetan Studies Library 10(5.) Leiden: Brill.
Ardussi, John, and Sonam Tobgay (ed.). 2008. *Written Treasures of Bhutan : Mirror of the Past and Bridge to the Future; Proceedings of the First International Conference on the Rich Scriptural Heritage of Bhutan.* Thimphu: National Library of Bhutan.
Aris, Michael. 1979. *Bhutan: The Early History of a Himalayan Kingdom.* Warminster: Aris & Phillips.
———. 1986. *Sources for the History of Bhutan.* Wiener Studien Zur Tibetologie Und Buddhismuskunde 14. Wien: Arbeitskreis für tibetische und buddhistische Studien, Universität Wien.
———. 1987. '"The Boneless Tongue": Alternative Voices from Bhutan in the Context of Lamaist Societies.' *Past & Present* (115) (May): 131–64.
———. 1994a. 'Introduction.' In *Bhutan: Aspects of Culture and Development*, ed. Michael Hutt, 7–23. Kiscadale Asia Research Series no. 5. Gartmore: Kiscadale.
———. 1994b. *The Raven Crown: The Origins of Buddhist Monarchy in Bhutan.* London: Serindia.
Aris, Michael, Susan S. Bean, Diana K. Myers, and Françoise Pommaret (ed.). 1994. *From the Land of the Thunder Dragon: Textile Arts of Bhutan.* London: Serindia.
Aris, Michael, and Samuel Davis. 1982. *Views of Medieval Bhutan: The Diary and Drawings of Samuel Davis 1783.* London: Serindia.
Aris, Michael, and Michael Hutt (eds.). 1994. *Bhutan: Aspects of Culture and Development.* Kiscadale Asia Research Series no. 5. Gartmore: Kiscadale.
Arya, Pasang. 1989. *History of Tibetan Medicine: Past and Present.* 1st ed. India: Self-Published. http://www.tibetanmedicine-edu.org/index.php/publications.
———. 2009. 'Traditional Medicine Materia Medica.' Tibetan Medicine Education Center. http://www.tibetanmedicine-edu.org/images/stories/pdf/materia_medica.pdf.
Aschoff, Jürgen C. 2003. 'The Spread of Tibetan Medicine.' In *Exile as Challenge: The Tibetan Diaspora*, ed. Dagmar Bernstorff and Hubertus von Welck. Hyderabad: Orient Blackswan.
Association of Social Anthropologists of the UK and the Commonwealth. 2010. 'Ethical Guidelines for Good Research Practice.' United Kingdom. http://www.theasa.org/ethics/guidelines.shtml.
Baer, Hans A. (ed.). 1987. *Encounters with Biomedicine: Case Studies in Medical Anthropology.* New York: Gordon and Breach Science Publishers.
———. 2001. *Biomedicine and Alternative Healing Systems in America: Issues of Class, Race, Ethnicity, and Gender.* Madison: University of Wisconsin Press.
Baer, Hans A., Merrill Singer, and Ida Susser. 2003. *Medical Anthropology and the World System.* Westport, CT: Greenwood Publishing Group.
Bajracharya, S. R., P. K. Mool, and B. R. Shrestha. 2007. *Impact of Climate Change on Himalayan Glaciers and Glacial Lakes: Case Studies on GLOF and Associated Hazards in Nepal and Bhutan.* Kathmandu: International Centre for Integrated Mountain Development (ICIMOD).

BBC. 2008. *Cordyceps: Attack of the Killer Fungi. Planet Earth.* London: BBC. http://www.youtube.com/watch?v=XuKjBIBBAL8&feature=youtube_gdata_player.

Bensky, Dan, Steven Clavey, and Erich Stöger. 2004. *Chinese Herbal Medicine: Materia Medica.* Seattle: USA: Eastland Press.

Bhutan Broadcast Service. 2011. 'Thimphu Hit by a Dearth of Drugs.' 1 November, online edition. http://www.bbs.bt/news/?p=3042.

———. 2012a. 'Bird Flu Outbreak Reported.' 4 January, online edition. http://www.bbs.bt/news/?p=8153.

———. 2012b. 'Traditional Medicines Seized from a Local Practitioner.' 17 April, online edition. http://www.bbs.bt/news/?p=12013.

———. 2012c. 'Wangduephodrang Dzong Completely Gutted.' 24J une, online edition. http://www.bbs.bt/news/?p=14477.

———. 2012d. '"Our Daughter Died because of Lack of Medicines": Parents.' 3 July, online edition. http://www.bbs.bt/news/?p=10398.

———. 2012e. '15th Is the Deadlines to Solve Drug Shortage.' 4 November, online edition. http://www.bbs.bt/news/?p=11793.

———. 2013. 'Punakha Hospital Fears Shortage of Drugs.' 6 April, online edition. http://www.bbs.bt/news/?p=21952.

Bhutan Observer. 2011. 'Allegedly Raping a 16-year-old Girl.' 9 March, online edition. http://bhutanobserver.bt/4740-bo-news-about-allegedly_raping_a_16yearold_girl_.aspx.

———. 2013. 'Larger Perspective on Prostitution.' 17 August, online edition. http://bhutanobserver.bt/5910-bo-news-about-larger_perspective__on_prostitution_.aspx.

Bisht, Medha. 2012. 'The Rupee Crunch and India-Bhutan Economic Engagement.' *IDSA Issue Briefs.* New Delhi: Institute for Defense Studies and Analyses. http://www.isn.ethz.ch/Digital-Library/Publications/Detail/?ots591=0c54e3b3-1e9c-be1e-2c24-a6a8c7060233&lng=en&id=150950.

Bodeker, Gerard, and Gemma Burford (eds.). 2007. *Traditional, Complementary and Alternative Medicine: Policy and Public Health Perspectives.* London: Imperial College Press.

Bodt, Timotheus. 2012. *Lamp Clarifying the History, Peoples, Languages and Traditions of Eastern Bhutan and Eastern Mon.* Wageningen: Monpasang Publications.

Boesi, Alessandro. 2003. 'The Dbyar Rtswa Dgun'Bu (Cordyceps Sinensis Berk.): An Important Trade Item for the Tibetan Population of the Lithang County, Sichuan Province, China.' *Tibet Journal* 283: 29–42.

———. 2006. 'Tibetan Herbal Medicine: Classification and Utilization of Natural Products Used as Materia Medica in Tibetan Traditional Medicine.' *Berbalgram* (71): 38–48.

———. 2007. 'The Nature of Tibetan Plant Nomenclature.' *Tibet Journal* 32: 3–28.

———. 2009. 'Cordyceps Sinensis Medicinal Fungus: Traditional Use among Tibetan People, Harvesting Techniques, and Modern Uses.' *Herbalgram* (83): 52–61.

———. 2015. *Tibetan Medicinal Plants: An Ancient Manuscript of the Tibetan Science of Healing.* Rome: Scienze e Lettere.

Bohler, Erik, and Staffan Bergström. 2008. 'Premature Weaning in East Bhutan: Only If Mother Is Pregnant Again.' *Journal of Biosocial Science* 27(3) (31 July): 253–65. doi:10.1017/S0021932000022781.

Bolsokhoeva, N. D. 1993. *Introduction to the Studies of Tibetan Medical Sources.* Kathmandu: Mandala Book Point.

Brooks, Jeremy. 2013. 'Avoiding the Limits to Growth: Gross National Happiness in Bhutan as a Model for Sustainable Development.' *Sustainability* 5(9) (26 August): 3640–64. doi:10.3390/su5093640.

Buch-Hansen, Mogens. 1997. 'Environment – A Liability and an Asset for Economic Development: Some Views on Environmental Protection with Economic Development in Bhutan.' *International Journal of Sustainable Development & World Ecology* 4(1): 17–27. doi:10.1080/13504509709469938.

Buncombe, Andrew, and Omar Waraich. 2011. 'No Smoking: Monk Jailed for Three Years in Bhutan.' *Independent* (3 May): online edition. http://www.independent. co.uk/news/world/asia/no-smoking-monk-jailed-for-three-years-in-bhutan-2232962.html.

Burri, Regula Valerie, and Josepch Dumit (eds.). 2007. *Biomedicine as Culture: Instrumental Practices, Technoscientific Knowledge, and New Modes of Life.* Oxon: Routledge.

Cai, Jingfeng, Byams-pa-phrin-las, Lei Wang, and Sde-srid Sańs-rgyas-rgya-mtsho. 2008. *Bod Lugs Gso Rig Rgyud-bźi'i Sman Thań [Tibetan Medical Thangka of the Four Medical Tantras].* Trans. and comp. of original ed. Byams-pa 'Phrin-las, Wang Lei. English trans. and annot. Cai Jingfeng. 2nd ed. Lhasa: Bod ljońs Mi-dmańs Dpe-skrun-khań.

Cannon, Paul F., Nigel L. Hywel-Jones, Norbert Maczey, Lungten Norbu, Tshitila, Tashi Samdup, and Phurba Lhendup. 2009. 'Steps towards Sustainable Harvest of Ophiocordyceps Sinensis in Bhutan.' *Biodiversity and Conservation* 18(9) (1 August): 2263–81. doi:10.1007/s10531-009-9587-5.

Cant, Sarah, and Ursula Sharma. 1996. *Complementary and Alternative Medicines: Knowledge in Practice.* London: Free Association Books.

———. 1999. *A New Medical Pluralism? Complementary Medicine, Doctors, Patients and the State.* London: Routledge.

Cawte, John. 1974. *Medicine Is the Law: Studies in Psychiatric Anthropology of Australian Tribal Societies.* Honolulu: University Press of Hawaii.

Centre for Bhutan Studies. 2004. *Wayo, Wayo – Voices from the Past.* Thimphu: Centre for Bhutan Studies.

Chen, Lincoln C., Arthur Kleinman, and Norma C. Ware (eds.). 1993. *Health and Social Change in International Perspective.* Boston: Dept. of Population and International Health, Harvard School of Public Health; distributed by Harvard University Press.

Choden, Kunzang. 2008a. 'The Malevolent Spirits of sTang Valley (Bumthang) – A Bhutanese Account.' *Revue d'Etudes Tibétaines* 15: 313–30.

———. 2008b. 'Literature in Bhutan.' In *Bhutan: Ways of Knowing,* ed. Frank Rennie and Robin Mason, 237–40. Charlotte, NC: Information Age Publishing.

———. 2009. *Tales in Colour and Other Stories.* New Delhi: Zubaan Books.

———. 2013. *Circle of Karma.* New Delhi: Zubaan Books.

Choden, Pema. 2009. 'Lang-dug: Herbal Steam Application.' *Menjong Sorig Journal* (2): 60–62.

Chupein, Thomas. 2010. 'Advancing Gross National Happiness: Spatially Targeted Development in Bhutan and the Importance of Rural Life.' MA Thesis. Boston: Harvard University.

Clifford, Terry. 1984. *The Diamond Healing: Tibetan Buddhist Medicine and Psychiatry.* York Beach, ME: Samuel Weiser, Inc.

———. 1994. *Tibetan Buddhist Medicine and Psychiatry: The Diamond Healing.* New Delhi: Motilal Banarsidass Publ.

Cohen, Lawrence. 1998. *No Aging in India: Alzheimer's, the Bad Family, and Other Modern Things.* Berkeley: University of California Press.

College of Natural Resources. 2008. 'Medicinal Plants and Aromatic Plants: An Overview.' In *Medicinal Aromatic Plants and Spices.* Thimphu: Royal University of Bhutan. http://cms.cnr.edu.bt/cms/medicinalaromaticDIP/?Chapter_1.

Collister, Peter. 1987. *Bhutan and the British*. London: Serindia Publications with Belitha Press.

Cooper, Amy Ellen. 2012. 'Vital Politics: Medicine and Citizenship in Venezuela.' PhD dissertation. Chicago: University of Chicago.

Coreil, Jeannine, and J. Dennis Mull (eds.). 1990. *Anthropology and Primary Health Care*. New York: Westview Press.

Craig, Sienna. 2005. 'Himalayan Healers in Transition: Professionalization, Identity and Conservation among Practitioners of Gso Ba Rig Pa in Nepal.' In *Himalayan Medicinal and Aromatic Plants, Balancing Use and Conservation: Proceedings of the Regional Workshop on Wise Practices and Experiential Learning in Conservation and Management of Himalayan Medicinal Plants, December 15–20, 2002, Kathmandu, Nepal*, ed. Yildiz Aumeeruddy-Thomas and Ministry of Forest and Soil Conservation, Nepal, 411–33. Kathmandu: Government of Nepal, Ministry of Forests and Soil Conservation.

———. 2007a. 'A Crisis of Confidence: A Comparison between Shifts in Tibetan Medical Education Nepal and Tibet.' In *Soundings in Tibetan Medicine: Anthropological and Historical Perspectives: PIATS 2003: Tibetan Studies: Proceedings of the Tenth Seminar of the International Association for Tibetan Studies, Oxford, 2003*, ed. Mona Schrempf, 127–154. Brill.

———. 2007b. 'Place and Professionalization: Navigating Amchi Identity in Nepal.' In *The World of Tibetan Medicine: Contemporary Trends in the Politics of Medical Knowledge and Practice*, ed. Laurent Pordié, 62–90. London: Routledge.

———. 2010. 'From Empowerments to Power Calculations: Notes on Efficacy, Value, and Method.' In *Medicine between Science and Religion*, ed. Vincanne Adams, Mona Schrempf, and Sienna Craig. London: Berghahn Books.

———. 2011. '"Good" Manufacturing by Whose Standards? Remaking Concepts of Quality, Safety, and Value in the Production of Tibetan Medicines.' *Anthropological Quarterly* 84(2): 331–78. doi:10.1353/anq.2011.0027.

———. 2012. *Healing Elements: Efficacy and the Social Ecologies of Tibetan Medicine*. Berkeley: University of California Press.

Craig, Sienna, and Vincanne Adams. 2008. 'Global Pharma in the Land of Snows: Tibetan Medicines, SARS, and Identity Politics across Nations.' *Asian Medicine* 4(1): 1–28. doi:10.1163/157342108X381205.

Craig, Sienna, Mingji Cuomo, Frances Garrett, and Mona Schrempf (eds.). 2010. *Studies of Medical Pluralism in Tibetan History and Society*. Proceedings of the 11th Seminar of the International Association for Tibetan Studies, PIATS, Bonn 2006. Andiast: International Institute for Tibetan and Buddhist Studies, GmbH.

Crandon-Malamud, Libbet. 1993. *From the Fat of Our Souls: Social Change, Political Process, and Medical Pluralism in Bolivia*. Berkeley: University of California Press.

Crigler, John F., and Victor A. Najjar. 1952. 'Congenital Familial Nonhemolytic Jaundice with Kernicterus.' *Pediatrics* 10(2) (1 August): 169–80.

Crins, Rieki. 2008. *Meeting the 'Other': Living in the Present; Gender and Sustainability in Bhutan*. Delft: Eburon.

Csordas, Thomas J. 1997a. *Language, Charisma, and Creativity: The Ritual Life of a Religious Movement*. Berkeley: University of California Press.

———. 1997b. *The Sacred Self*. Berkeley: University of California Press.

———. 2002. *Body/Meaning/Healing*. Basingstoke: Palgrave Macmillan.

Dale, Rice, and Steven Schaefer. 2004. *Endoscopic Paranasal Sinus Surgery*. Philadelphia: Lippincott Williams & Wilkins.

Das, Veena, and Ranendra Das. 2006. 'Pharmaceuticals in Urban Ecologies: The Register of the Local.' In *Global Pharmaceuticals: Ethics, Markets, Practices*, ed. Adriana

Petryna, Andrew Lakoff, and Arthur Kleinman. Durham, 171–205. NC: Duke University Press.

Dash, Bhagwan. 1991. *Positive Health in Tibetan Medicine: Based on Sman-'tsho-Ba'i Mdo (Vaidya-Jīva-Sūtra)*. Indian Medical Science Series 13. Delhi: Sri Satguru Publications.

Deki, Tashi. 2012. 'Pharmacies Also Bear the Brunt of Drug Shortage.' *The Bhutanese*, 14 March. http://www.thebhutanese.bt/ pharmacies-also-bear-the-brunt-of-drug-shortage/.

DeLanda, Manuel. 2006. *A New Philosophy of Society: Assemblage Theory and Social Complexity*. New York: Continuum International Publishing Group.

Deleuze, Gilles, and Félix Guattari. 2004. *A Thousand Plateaus: Capitalism and Schizophrenia*. New York: Continuum International Publishing Group.

Desjarlais, Robert, Leon Eisenberg, Byron Good, and Arthur Kleinman (eds.). 1995. *World Mental Health: Problems and Priorities in Low-Income Countries*. Oxford: Oxford University Press.

Desjarlais, Robert R. 2003. *Sensory Biographies: Lives and Deaths among Nepal's Yolmo Buddhists*. Ethnographic Studies in Subjectivity 2. Berkeley: University of California Press.

Diemberger, Hildegard. 2005. 'Female Oracles in Modern Tibet.' In *Women in Tibet*, ed. Janet Gyatso and Hanna Havnevik, 113–168. New York: Columbia University Press.

Diemberger, Hildegard, Kirsten Hastrup, Simon Schaffer, Charles F. Kennel, David Sneath, Michael Bravo, Hans-F. Graf, et al. 2012. 'Communicating Climate Knowledge.' *Current Anthropology* 53(2) (April): 226–44. doi:10.1086/665033.

Dogra, R. C. 1990. *Bhutan*. World Bibliographic Series. Santa Barbara, CA: Clio Press.

Dönden, Yeshi. 1986. *Health through Balance: An Introduction to Tibetan Medicine*. Trans. and ed. Jeffrey Hopkins. 1st South Asian ed. Ithaca, NY: Snow Lion Publications.

———. 2000. *Healing from the Source: The Science and Lore of Tibetan Medicine*. Trans. and ed. Alan Wallace. Ithaca, NY: Snow Lion Publications.

Dorji, C. T. 1997. *An Introduction to Bhutanese Languages*. New Delhi: Vikas.

———. 2004. *Sources of Bhutanese History*. New Delhi: Prominent Publishers, Distributor, Chengay Dorji.

Dorji, Chencho. 2009. 'Health Services in Bhutan.' Thimphu, Bhutan: Centre for Bhutan Studies.

Dorji, Kinley. 2002. 'Five Prostitutes Arrested.' *Kuensel* Online, 16 August. http://www.kuenselonline.com.

Dorji, Rigzin. 1987. *Significance of Chibdrel, Serdeng and Zhugdrel Ceremonies*. Thimphu: Special Commission.

Dorji, Tandin. 2002. 'The Lha "Bod": An Invocation Ritual in Sbe Nag (Western Bhutan).' In *Territory and Identity in Tibet and the Himalayas, Tibetan Studies in Honour of Anne-Marie Blondeau, Proceedings of the 9th IATS, Leiden 2000*, ed. K. Buffetrille and H. Diemberger, 179–194. Leiden: Brill Tibetan Studies Library.

———. 2004. 'The Spider, the Piglet and the Vital Principle: A Popular Ritual for Restoring the Srog.' In *The Spider and the Piglet: Proceedings of the First International Seminar on Bhutan Studies*, ed. Karma Ura and Sonam Kinga, 598–97. Thimphu: Centre for Bhutan Studies.

———. 2007. 'Acquiring Power: A Modality of Becoming a Pawo (dpa 'bo).' In *Bhutan: Traditions and Changes; PIATS 2003: Tibetan Studies: Proceedings of the Tenth Seminar of the International Association for Tibetan Studies, Oxford, 2003*, ed. John Ardussi and Françoise Pommaret. Brill's Tibetan Studies Library 10(5). Leiden: Brill.

———. 2008. 'The Cult of Radrap (Ra Dgra), "Nep" of Wangdue Phodrang (Bhutan).' *Revue d'Etudes Tibétaines* 15: 357–70.

———. 2009. 'Ritualizing Story: A Way to Heal Malady.' *Journal of Bhutan Studies* 20.

Dorji, Ugyen. 2007. 'Wild Harvesting of Medicinal Plants in Lingzhi, Bhutan: An Ethnobotanical Approach to Understanding Its Social and Ecological Impacts and the Prospects for Sustainable Extraction.' Master of Science by Research in Ethnobiology, UK. University of Kent at Canterbury.

———. 2012. 'Cordyceps Prices Hits All-Time High, but Yield Is Low in Few Places.' *The Bhutanese*, online edition. http://www.thebhutanese.bt/ cordyceps-prices-hits-all-time-high-but-yield-is-low-in-few-places/.

Driem, George van. 1991. 'Guide to Official Dzongkha Romanization.' Thimphu: Royal Government of Bhutan. http://www.himalayanlanguages.org/files/driem/ pdfs/1991Romanization.pdf.

———. 2004. 'Endangered Languages of Bhutan and Sikkim: South Bodish Languages.' In *Encyclopedia of the World's Endangered Languages*, ed. Christopher Moseley. New York: Routledge.

Driem, George van, and Karma Tshering. 1998. *Dzongkha*. Leiden: Research CNWS, School of Asian, African, and Amerindian Studies.

Drug Regulatory Authority. 2006. 'Guidelines for Application for Registration of Medicinal Products.' Thimphu: Drug Regulatory Authority, Royal Government of Bhutan. http://www.health.gov.bt/downloads/draRegisGuidenew.pdf.

———. 2012. 'Bhutan Medicines Rules and Regulation 2012.' Thimphu: Drug Regulatory Authority, Royal Government of Bhutan. http://www.dra.gov.bt/images/ bmrr%202012.pdf.

———. 2013a. 'Drug Regulatory Authority Website.' http://www.dra.gov.bt/.

———. 2013b. 'Essential Drug List.' http://www.dra.gov.bt/index.php/ essential-drug-list.

———. 2013c. 'Registration of Medicinal Products 2nd Edition, 2013.' Thimphu: Drug Regulatory Authority, Royal Government of Bhutan. http://www.dra.gov.bt/images/ Guidelines%20for%20Registration%20of%20Medicinal%20Products.pdf.

Drugs, Vaccines and Equipment Division. 2013. 'Drugs, Vaccines and Equipment Division.' http://www.dved.gov.bt/.

Duncan, Amanda Sarah. 2008. 'Buddhism, Biomedicine, and Happiness in the Healing Traditions of Contemporary Bhutan.' MA thesis. University of Alberta.

Dzongkha Development Commission. 1997. *Samples for Geographical Names of Bhutan in Dzongkha and Romanized Dzongkha with Brief Guidelines*. Thimphu: Dzongkha Development Commission.

———. 2010. *English-Dzongkha Pocket Dictionary*. Rev. ed. Thimphu: Dzongkha Development Commission.

———. 2012. *English-Dzongkha Agricultural Terminology*. Thimphu: Dzongkha Development Commission. http://www.dzongkha.gov.bt/publications/ Publications_2011-2012.en.html#Agri-Term.

Eden, Ashley, and R. B. Pemberton. 1865. *Political Missions to Bootan: Comprising the Reports of the Hon'ble Ashley Eden, 1864, R.B. Pemberton, 1837, 1838, with W. Griffiths's Journal and the Account by Kishen Kant Bose*. Calcutta: Printed at the Bengal Secretariat Office.

Ernst, Waltraud (ed.). 2002. *Plural Medicine, Tradition and Modernity, 1800–2000*. Studies in the Social History of Medicine 13. London: Routledge.

Ethnologue. 2013. 'Dzongkha.' http://www.ethnologue.com/language/dzo.

Farmer, Paul. 2001. *Infections and Inequalities: The Modern Plagues*. Berkeley: University of California Press.

Farmer, Paul. 2004. *Pathologies of Power*. Berkeley: University of California Press.

Fischer, Tim, and Tshering Tashi. 2009. *From Jesuits to Jetsetters: Bold Bhutan Beckons; Inhaling Gross National Happiness*. Brisbane: Copyright Pub. Co.

Fiumara, Karen, and Samuel Z. Goldhaber. 2009. 'A Patient's Guide to Taking Coumadin/Warfarin.' *Circulation* 119(8) (3 March): e220–22. doi:10.1161/CIRCULATIONAHA.108.803957.

Gallenkamp, Marian. 2011. 'The History of Institutional Change in the Kingdom of Bhutan: A Tale of Vision, Resolve, and Power.' Heidelberg Papers in South Asian and Comparative Politics. Working Paper No. 61. http://archiv.ub.uni-heidelberg.de/volltextserver/volltexte/2011/12042/pdf/Heidelberg_Papers_61_Gallenkamp.pdf.

Gardiner, Chris, Karen Williams, Ian J. Mackie, Samuel J. Machin, and Hannah Cohen. 2005. 'Patient Self-Testing Is a Reliable and Acceptable Alternative to Laboratory INR Monitoring.' *British Journal of Haematology* 128(2): 242–47. doi:10.1111/j.1365-2141.2004.05300.x.

Garrett, Frances. 2008. *Religion, Medicine and the Human Embryo in Tibet*. New York: Routledge.

Gayley, Holly. 2007. 'Patterns in the Ritual Dissemination of Padma Gling Pa's Treasures.' In *Bhutan: Traditions and Changes; PIATS 2003: Tibetan Studies: Proceedings of the Tenth Seminar of the International Association for Tibetan Studies, Oxford, 2003*, ed. John Ardussi and Françoise Pommaret. Brill's Tibetan Studies Library 10(5). Leiden: Brill.

Gerke, Barbara. 2007. 'Engaging the Subtle Body: Re-Approaching Bla Rituals in the Himalayas.' In *Soundings in Tibetan Medicine: Anthropological and Historical Perspectives: PIATS 2003: Tibetan Studies: Proceedings of the Tenth Seminar of the International Association for Tibetan Studies, Oxford, 2003*, ed. Mona Schrempf, 191–22. Leiden: Brill.

———. 2011. *Long Lives and Untimely Deaths: Life-Span Concepts and Longevity Practices among Tibetans in the Darjeeling Hills, India*. Leiden: Brill.

Germano, David, and Nicholas Tournadre. 2003. 'THL Simplified Phonetic Transcription of Standard Tibetan.' http://www.thlib.org/reference/transliteration/#!essay=/thl/phonetics/.

Good, Byron. 1994. *Medicine, Rationality, and Experience: An Anthropological Perspective*. The Lewis Henry Morgan Lectures 1990. Cambridge: Cambridge University Press.

Good, Byron J., Michael M. J. Fischer, Sarah S. Willen, and Mary-Jo DelVecchio Good (eds.). 2010. *A Reader in Medical Anthropology: Theoretical Trajectories, Emergent Realities*. Oxford: John Wiley & Sons.

Goroll, Allan H., and Albert G. Mulley. 2012. *Primary Care Medicine: Office Evaluation and Management of the Adult Patient*. Philadelphia: Lippincott Williams & Wilkins.

Government of Great Britain. 1908. 'Sketch Map of Bhutan, Sikkim and a Portion of Tibet.' Simla: Intelligence Branch.

Griffiths, Marcia. 1990. 'Using Anthropological Techniques in Program Design: Successful Nutrition in Indonesia.' In *Anthropology and Primary Health Care*, ed. Jeannine Coreil and J. Dennis Mull. New York: Westview Press.

Gross National Happiness Commission. 2013. 'FAQs on GNH.' Thimphu. http://www.gnhc.gov.bt/wp-content/uploads/2013/04/GNH-FAQs-pdf.pdf.

Grujic, Djordje, Isabelle Coutand, Bodo Bookhagen, Stéphane Bonnet, Ann Blythe, and Chris Duncan. 2006. 'Climatic Forcing of Erosion, Landscape, and Tectonics in the Bhutan Himalayas.' *Geology* 34(10) (1 October): 801–4. doi:10.1130/G22648.1.

Gueye, Cara Smith, and Thinley Yangzom. 2011. 'APMEN Report: Bhutan and Cross-Border Malaria.' Asia Pacific Malaria Elimination Network. http://apmen.org/storage/country-partner/APMEN%20XBorder%20Report%20May2011.pdf.

Gupta, Akhil, and James Ferguson. 1997. *Culture, Power, Place: Explorations in Critical Anthropology*. Durham, NC: Duke University Press.

Gurung, Tulsi. 2008. 'Organic Farming.' In *Bhutan: Ways of Knowing*, ed. Frank Rennie and Robin Mason, 205–10. Charlotte, NC: Information Age Publishing.

Gyal, Yangbum. 2006. *Tibetan Medical Dietary Book*. Vol. 1: *Potency & Preparation of Vegetables*. Trans. Tenzin Namdul. Dharamsala: Clinical Research Dept., Men-Tsee-Khang.

Hamilton, Alan C. 2004. 'Medicinal Plants, Conservation and Livelihoods.' *Biodiversity & Conservation* 13(8) (1 July): 1477–1517. doi:10.1023/B:BIOC.0000021333.23413.42.

Hansen, Thor. 2013. 'Neonatal Jaundice.' *Medscape* (June 11). http://emedicine.medscape.com/article/974786-overview.

Harner, Michael J. 1980. *The Way of the Shaman: A Guide to Power and Healing*. San Francisco: Harper & Row.

Harrison, Vincent. 2008. *The Newborn Baby*. Cape Town: Juta and Company Ltd.

Healy, Adriana. 2006. 'The New Medical Oikumene.' In *Global Pharmaceuticals: Ethics, Markets, Practices*, ed. Andrew Lakoff, Adriana Petryna, and Arthur Kleinman, 61–84. Durham, NC: Duke University Press.

Hemmings, Colin P. 2005. 'Rethinking Medical Anthropology: How Anthropology Is Failing Medicine.' *Anthropology & Medicine* 12(2): 91. doi:10.1080/13648470500139841.

Heywood, V. 2000. 'Management and Sustainability of the Resource Base for Medicinal Plants.' In *Medicinal Utilization of Wild Species: Challenge for Man and Nature in the New Millennium*, ed. S. Honnef and R. Melisch. Hanover: WWF Germany/TRAFFIC Europe-Germany, EXPO 2000.

Hickman, Katie. 1987. *Dreams of the Peaceful Dragon: A Journey through Bhutan*. London: Gollancz.

Hofer, Theresia. 2011. 'Tibetan Medicine on the Margins: Twentieth Century Transformations of the Traditions of Sowa Rigpa in Central Tibet.' PhD thesis.. London: University of College London.

———. 2012. *'The Inheritance of Change': Transmission and Practice of Tibetan Medicine in Ngamring*. Vienna: Vienna Studies in Tibetology and Buddhism.

Holbrook, Anne M., Jennifer A. Pereira, Renee Labiris, Heather McDonald, James D. Douketis, Mark Crowther, and Philip S. Wells. 2005. 'Systematic Overview of Warfarin and Its Drug and Food Interactions.' *Archives of Internal Medicine* 165(10) (23 May): 1095–106. doi:10.1001/archinte.165.10.1095.

Hollan, Douglas. 1994. 'Suffering and the Work of Culture: A Case of Magical Poisoning in Toraja.' *American Ethnologist* 21(1) (February): 74–87.

Huber, Toni. 2013. 'The Iconography of G Shen Priests in the Ethnographic Context of the Extended Eastern Himalayas, and Reflections on the Development of Bon Religion.' In *Nepalica-Tibetica: Festgabe for Christoph Cüppers*, ed. Franz-Karl Ehrhard and Petra Maurer, 1:263–94. Andiast: International Institute for Tibetan and Buddhist Studies.

———. 2014. 'Hunting for the Cure: A Bon Healing Narrative from Eastern Bhutan.' In *Tibetan and Himalayan Healing: An Anthology for Anthony Aris*, ed. Charles Ramble and Ulrike Rösler, 369–80. Kathmandu: Vajra Books.

Hutt, Michael. 1994. *Bhutan: Perspectives on Conflict and Dissent*. Kiscadale Asia Research Series 3. Gartmore: Kiscadale.

Institute of Language and Culture Studies, UNESCO, and Royal University of Bhutan. 2006. 'Bhutan Cultural Atlas.' http://www.bhutanculturalatlas.org/.

Isbister, Geoffrey K., L. Peter Hackett, and Ian M. Whyte. 2003. 'Intentional Warfarin Overdose.' *Therapeutic Drug Monitoring* 25(6) (December): 715–22.

Iyer, Venkat. 2008. 'Defamation Law in Bhutan: Some Reflections.' *Journal of Bhutan Studies* 18 (Summer): 82–94.

Jamphel, Kinga. 2008. 'Scope and Challenges of the Bhutanese Traditional Medicine in the 21st Century.' *Menjong Sorig Journal* (1): 94–98.

Janes, Craig R. 1995. 'The Transformations of Tibetan Medicine.' *Medical Anthropology Quarterly* 9(1): 6–39. doi:10.1525/maq.1995.9.1.02a00020.

Janzen, John M. 1982. *The Quest for Therapy: Medical Pluralism in Lower Zaire*. Berkeley: University of California Press.

Jensen, Torben Elgaard, and Brit Ross Winthereik. 2005. 'Book Review: *The Body Multiple: Ontology in Medical Practice*.' *Acta Sociologica* 48(3) (1 September): 266–68. doi:10.1177/000169930504800309.

Johannessen, Helle. 2006. 'Introduction: Body and Self in Medical Pluralism.' In *Multiple Medical Realities: Patients and Healers in Biomedical, Alternative, and Traditional Medicine*, ed. Helle Johannessen and Imre Lazar, 1–20. New York: Berghahn Books.

Karmay, Samten Gyaltsen. 1998. *The Arrow and the Spindle: Studies in History, Myths, Rituals and Beliefs in Tibet*. Kathmandu: Mandala Book Point.

Kennedy, D. W. 1985. 'Functional Endoscopic Sinus Surgery: Technique.' *Archives of Otolaryngology (Chicago: 1960)*, 111(10) (October): 643–649.

Kim, Chŏngho. 2003. *Korean Shamanism: The Cultural Paradox*. Farnham: Ashgate Publishing, Ltd.

Kim, Jim Yong, Alec Irwin, Joyce Millen, and John Gershman (eds.). 2000. *Dying for Growth: Global Inequality and the Health of the Poor*. Monroe, ME: Common Courage Press.

Kinga, Sonam. 2008. 'Reciprocal Exchange and Community Vitality: The Case of Gortshom Village in Eastern Bhutan.' In *Towards Global Transformation: Proceedings of the Third International Conference on Gross National Happiness*, 31–64. Thimphu: The Centre for Bhutan Studies.

———. 2009. *Polity, Kingship and Democracy: A Biography of the Bhutanese State*. Thimphu: Royal Government of Bhutan.

Kleinman, Arthur. 1981. *Patients and Healers in the Context of Culture*. Berkeley: University of California Press.

Kohli, Manorama. 1982. *India and Bhutan: A Study in Interrelations, 1772–1910*. New Delhi: Munshiram Manoharlal.

Kuensel Online. 2013. 'From The Readers.' *Kuensel* Online. http://www.kuenselonline.com/forums/forum/from-the-readers/.

Kumar, Vinay, Abul K. Abbas, and Jon C. Aster. 2012. *Robbins Basic Pathology, 9th Edition*. Philadelphia: Elsevier Health Sciences.

Kuyakanon Knapp, Riamsara. 2015. 'Environmental Modernity in Bhutan: Entangled Landscapes, Buddhist Narratives and Inhabiting the Land.' PhD Thesis. Cambridge: University of Cambridge.

Lambert, Helen, and Maryon McDonald (eds.). 2009. *Social Bodies*. New York: Berghahn Books.

Latour, Bruno. 1987. *Science in Action: How to Follow Scientists and Engineers Through Society*. Cambridge, MA: Harvard University Press.

———. 1991. *We Have Never Been Modern*. Cambridge, MA: Harvard University Press.

———. 2005. *Reassembling the Social: An Introduction to Actor-Network-Theory.* Illustrated ed. Oxford: Oxford University Press.

Leslie, Charles M. (ed.). 1976. *Asian Medical Systems: A Comparative Study.* Berkeley: University of California Press.

———. 1978. *Theoretical Foundations for the Comparative Study of Medical Systems.* Oxford: Pergamon.

Leslie, Charles M., and Allan Young (eds.). 1992. *Paths to Asian Medical Knowledge.* Berkeley: University of California Press.

Leslie, Jacques. 2013. 'A Torrent of Consequence.' *World Policy Journal* (Summer). http://www.worldpolicy.org/journal/summer2013/torrent-consequences.

Lewis, Gilbert. 2000. *A Failure of Treatment.* Oxford Studies in Social and Cultural Anthropology. Oxford: Oxford University Press.

Leytho. 2009. 'Diagnostic Methods in Traditional Medicine System.' *Menjong Sorig Journal* (2): 63–69.

Lhamo, Namgay. 2010. 'Attitude of Bhutanese People on Traditional Medicine (gSoba-Rig-Pa): A Preliminary Study.' *Menjong Sorig Journal* (3): 32–46.

———. 2011. 'Health Seeking Behavior Relating to Sowa Rigpa in Bhutan.' Thimphu: National Institute of Traditional Medicine, Royal University of Bhutan.

Lhamo, Namgay, and Sabine Nebel. 2011. 'Perceptions and Attitudes of Bhutanese People on Sowa Rigpa, Traditional Bhutanese Medicine: A Preliminary Study from Thimphu.' *Journal of Ethnobiology and Ethnomedicine* 7: 3, doi:10.1186/1746-4269-7-3.

Lim, Francis Khek Gee. 2008. *Imagining the Good Life: Negotiating Culture and Development in Nepal Himalaya.* Leiden: Brill.

Lock, Margaret M., and Deborah R. Gordon (ed.). 1988. *Biomedicine Examined.* London: Springer.

Lock, Margaret M., and Vinh-Kim Nguyen. 2010. *An Anthropology of Biomedicine.* Chichester: Wiley-Blackwell.

Lockerbie, Stacy, and D. Ann Herring. 2009. 'Global Panic, Local Repercussions: Economic and Nutritional Effects of Bird Flu in Vietnam.' In *Anthropology and Public Health: Bridging Differences in Culture and Society,* ed. Robert Hahn and Marcia C. Inhorn, 566–87. 2nd ed. New York: Oxford University Press.

Lorway, Robert, Gampo Dorji, Janet Bradley, B. M. Ramesh, Shajy Isaac, and James Blanchard. 2011. 'The Drayang Girls of Thimphu: Sexual Network Formation, Transactional Sex and Emerging Modernities in Bhutan.' *Culture, Health & Sexuality* 13 (sup2) (December): S293–S308. doi:10.1080/13691058.2011.607243.

Lubetsky, A., E. Dekel-Stern, A. Chetrit, F. Lubin, and H. Halkin. 1999. 'Vitamin K Intake and Sensitivity to Warfarin in Patients Consuming Regular Diets.' *Thrombosis and Haemostasis* 81(3) (March): 396–99.

Maisels, M. J. 2005. 'Jaundice.' In *Avery's Neonatology: Pathophysiology & Management of the Newborn,* ed. Mhairi G. MacDonald, Mary M. K. Seshia, and Martha D. Mullett, 768–846. 6th ed. Philadelphia: Lippincott Williams & Wilkins.

———. 2006. 'Neonatal Jaundice.' *Pediatrics in Review* 27(12) (1 December): 443–54. doi:10.1542/pir.27-12-443.

Maisels, M. J., and J. F. Watchko. 2000. *Neonatal Jaundice.* Reading: Harwood Academic.

Malkki, Liisa. 1992. 'National Geographic: The Rooting of Peoples and the Territorialization of National Identity Among Scholars and Refugees.' *Cultural Anthropology* 7(1): 24–44. doi:10.1525/can.1992.7.1.02a00030.

Martin, Emily. 2001. *The Woman in the Body: A Cultural Analysis of Reproduction.* Boston: Beacon Press.

McDonald, Maryon. 2012. 'Medical Anthropology and Anthropological Studies of Science.' In *Companion to the Anthropology of Europe*, ed. U. Kockel, M. Nic Craith, and J. Frykman. Oxford: Wiley-Blackwell.

McKay, Alex. 2004. 'British-Indian Medical Service Officers in Bhutan, 1905–1947: A Historical Outline.' In *The Spider and the Piglet: Proceedings of the First International Seminar on Bhutan Studies*, ed. Karma Ura and Sonam Kinga, 137–59. Thimphu: Centre for Bhutan Studies.

———. 2007. *Their Footprints Remain: Biomedical Beginnings across the Indo-Tibetan Frontier*. Amsterdam: Amsterdam University Press.

McKay, Alex, and Dorji Wangchuk. 2005. 'Traditional Medicine in Bhutan.' *Asian Medicine* 1(1) (January): 204–18. doi:10.1163/157342105777996737.

McKechnie, Rosemary. 1999. 'Identifying Boundaries in Care: Human Immunodeficiency Virus and Men Who Have Sex with Men.' In *Extending the Boundaries of Care: Medical Ethics and Caring Practices*, ed. Tamara Kohn and Rosemary McKechnie, 19–48. Oxford: Berg Publishers.

Melgaard, Bjorn, and Tandi Dorji. 2012. *Medical History of Bhutan*. Thimphu: Centre for Research Initiatives.

Menjong Sorig Pharmaceuticals. 2008a. *Monograph on Medicinal Plants of Bhutan*. Vol. 1. Thimphu: Pharmaceutical and Research Unit, Institute for Traditional Medical Services.

———. 2008b. *Monograph on Medicinal Plants of Bhutan*. Vol. 2. Thimphu: Pharmaceutical and Research Unit, Institute for Traditional Medical Services.

———. 2013. 'Formulary.' Internal document. Menjong Sorig Pharmaceuticals.

Merleau-Ponty, Maurice. 2002. *Phenomenology of Perception*. Routledge Classics. London: Routledge.

Meyer, Fernand. 1981. *Gso-ba rig-pa, le système médical tibétain*. Paris: Editions du Centre national de la recherche scientifique.

———. 1990. 'Théorie et Pratique de L'examen Des Pouls Dans Un Chapitre Du rGyud-bzhi.' In *Indo-Tibetan Studies: Papers in Honour and Appreciation of Professor David L. Snellgrove's Contribution in Indo-Tibetan Studies*, ed. T. Skorupski, 209–56. Tring: Institute of Buddhist Studies.

———. 1997. 'Theory and Practice of Tibetan Medicine.' In *Oriental Medicine: An Illustrate Guide to the Asian Arts of Healing*. Boston: Shambala Publications.

Micozzi, Marc S. 2013. *Vital Healing: Energy, Mind and Spirit in Traditional Medicines of India, Tibet and the Middle East – Middle Asia*. Philadelphia: Singing Dragon.

Miller, Daniel. 2005. 'Materiality: An Introduction.' In *Materiality*, ed. Daniel Miller, 1–50. Durham, NC: Duke University Press.

Miller, Suellen, Phuoc V. Le, Sienna Craig, Vincanne Adams, Carrie Tudor, Sonam Nyima, et al. 2007. 'How to Make Consent Informed: Possible Lessons from Tibet.' *IRB: Ethics and Human Research* 29(6) (1 November): 7–14. doi:10.2307/30033249.

Ministry of Agriculture and Forests. 2010. 'Action Taken on 25 February 2010 to Rapidly Contain Bird Flu Outbreak at Rinchending and Pasakha, Phuentsholing.' Thimphu: Ministry of Agriculture and Forests, Royal Government of Bhutan. http://www.moa.gov.bt/ncah/admin/outbreakFiles/outbreak2010-02-268tu5879hj.pdf.

———. 2013. 'Bhutan RNR Statistics: 2012.' Thimphu: Policy and Planning Division, Ministry of Agriculture and Forests, Royal Government of Bhutan.

Ministry of Finance. 2013. 'National Budget Report.' Thimphu: Ministry of Finance, Royal Government of Bhutan. http://www.mof.gov.bt/publication/files/pub8pp7779lm.pdf.

Ministry of Health. 1986. 'Annual Health Bulletin 1986.' Thimphu: Ministry of Health, Royal Government of Bhutan.

———. 1987. 'Annual Health Bulletin 1987.' Thimphu: Ministry of Health, Royal Government of Bhutan.

———. 1988. 'Annual Health Bulletin 1988.' Thimphu: Ministry of Health, Royal Government of Bhutan.

———. 1989. 'Annual Health Bulletin 1989.' Thimphu: Ministry of Health, Royal Government of Bhutan.

———. 1990. 'Annual Health Bulletin 1990.' Thimphu: Ministry of Health, Royal Government of Bhutan.

———. 1991. 'Annual Health Bulletin 1991.' Thimphu: Ministry of Health, Royal Government of Bhutan.

———. 1992. 'Annual Health Bulletin 1992.' Thimphu: Ministry of Health, Royal Government of Bhutan.

———. 1993. 'Annual Health Bulletin 1993.' Thimphu: Ministry of Health, Royal Government of Bhutan.

———. 1994. 'Annual Health Bulletin 1994.' Thimphu: Ministry of Health, Royal Government of Bhutan.

———. 1995. 'Annual Health Bulletin 1995.' Thimphu: Ministry of Health, Royal Government of Bhutan.

———. 1996. 'Annual Health Bulletin 1996.' Thimphu: Ministry of Health, Royal Government of Bhutan.

———. 1997. 'Annual Health Bulletin 1997.' Thimphu: Ministry of Health, Royal Government of Bhutan.

———. 1998. 'Annual Health Bulletin 1998.' Thimphu: Ministry of Health, Royal Government of Bhutan.

———. 1999. 'Annual Health Bulletin 1999.' Thimphu: Ministry of Health, Royal Government of Bhutan.

———. 2000a. 'Annual Health Bulletin 2000.' Thimphu: Ministry of Health, Royal Government of Bhutan.

———. 2000b. 'National Health Survey: 2000.' Thimphu: Ministry of Health, Royal Government of Bhutan. http://www.health.gov.bt/healthSurvey/ nationalHealthSurvey2000.pdf.

———. 2001. 'Annual Health Bulletin 2001.' Thimphu: Ministry of Health, Royal Government of Bhutan.

———. 2002a. 'Annual Health Bulletin 2002.' Thimphu: Ministry of Health, Royal Government of Bhutan.

———. 2002b. The Medical and Health Council Act. http://www.health.gov.bt/ downloads.php.

———. 2003. 'Annual Health Bulletin 2003.' Thimphu: Ministry of Health, Royal Government of Bhutan.

———. 2004. 'Annual Health Bulletin 2004.' Thimphu: Ministry of Health, Royal Government of Bhutan.

———. 2006a. 'Annual Health Bulletin 2006.' Thimphu: Ministry of Health, Royal Government of Bhutan.

———. 2006b. 'Annual Health Bulletin 2007.' Thimphu: Ministry of Health, Royal Government of Bhutan.

———. 2007. 'Health Sector Review.' Thimphu: Ministry of Health, Royal Government of Bhutan.

———. 2008a. 'Annual Health Bulletin 2008.' Thimphu: Ministry of Health, Royal Government of Bhutan.

Ministry of Health. 2008b. 'History of HIV/AIDS and STDs.' Thimphu: Ministry of Health, Royal Government of Bhutan. http://www.health.gov.bt/doph/cdd/ hivHistory.pdf.

———. 2009. 'Annual Health Bulletin 2009.' Thimphu: Ministry of Health, Royal Government of Bhutan.

———. 2010. 'Annual Health Bulletin 2010.' Thimphu: Ministry of Health, Royal Government of Bhutan.

———. 2011a. 'Annual Health Bulletin 2011.' Thimphu: Ministry of Health, Royal Government of Bhutan.

———. 2011b. 'National Health Policy.' Thimphu: Ministry of Health, Royal Government of Bhutan.

———. 2011c. 'Traditional Healers Training Guideline.' Thimphu: Ministry of Health, Royal Government of Bhutan.

———. 2011d. 'Mapping of Health Infrastructures and Indicators Using Geographic Information System.' Thimphu: Ministry of Health, Royal Government of Bhutan.

———. 2011e. 'National Health Accounts: Tracking Resources in Health, 2009–2010.' Thimphu: Ministry of Health, Royal Government of Bhutan. http://www.health.gov. bt/publications/BNHS/bnhs200910.pdf.

———. 2012. 'Annual Health Bulletin 2012.' Thimphu: Ministry of Health, Royal Government of Bhutan.

———. 2013a. 'Annual Health Bulletin 2013.' Thimphu: Ministry of Health, Royal Government of Bhutan.

———. 2013b. 'Sowei Lhenkhag – Ministry of Health.' http://www.health.gov.bt/index.php.

Ministry of Information and Communications. 2011. 'Annual Info-Comm and Transport Statistical Bulletin.' Ministry of Information and Communications, Royal Government of Bhutan. http://www.moic.gov.bt/Statistical/annual%20 infocomm%20and%20transport%20statistical%20bulletin.pdf.

Ministry of Labour and Human Resources. 2012. 'Labour Force Survey Report: 2012.' Thimphu: Ministry of Labour and Human Resources, Royal Government of Bhutan.

Misra, Harikesh N. 1988. *Bhutan, Problems and Policies*. New Delhi: Heritage Publishers.

Mol, Annemarie. 2003. *The Body Multiple: Ontology in Medical Practice*. Durham, NC: Duke University Press.

———. 2008. *The Logic of Care*. London: Routledge.

Namgyel, Tenzin. 2013a. 'A Kilo of Cordyceps Fetches More than a Million.' *Kuensel* Online, 22 July. http://www.kuenselonline.com.

———. 2013b. 'What Determines Price of Cordyceps?' *Kuensel* Online, 24 July. http:// www.kuenselonline.com.

———. 2013c. 'Cordyceps Collectors Are Back for P-Day.' *Kuensel* Online, 7 November. http://www.kuenselonline.com.

Napolitano, Valentina, and David Pratten. 2007. 'Michel de Certeau: Ethnography and the Challenge of Plurality.' *Social Anthropology* 15(1): 1–12. doi:10.1111/j.1469-8676.2007.00005.x.

National Assembly of Bhutan. 1958. 'Resolutions Adopted During the 11th Session of the National Assembly of Bhutan on the 14th Day of the 9th Month of the Earth Dog Year.' Thimphu: National Assembly of Bhutan

———. 2003. 'The Medicines Act of the Kingdon of Bhutan.' Thimphu: National Assembly of Bhutan

National Institute of Health and Care Excellence. 2010. 'Neonatal Jaundice (CG98).' https://www.nice.org.uk/guidance/cg98?unlid=4206564752016101012415

National Institute of Traditional Medicine (ed.). 2013. *Menjong Sorig Journal*. http:// www.nitm.edu.bt/?page_id=165.

National Statistics Bureau. 2005. 'Socio-Economic and Demographic Indicators.' Thimphu: National Statistics Bureau, Royal Government of Bhutan. http://www. nsb.gov.bt/publication/files/pub9zy4063xj.pdf.

———. 2007. 'Bhutan Living Standards Survey.' Thimphu: National Statistics Bureau, Royal Government of Bhutan.

———. 2012. 'Statistical Yearbook.' Thimphu: National Statistics Bureau, Royal Government of Bhutan. http://www.nsb.gov.bt/publication/files/pub10pp3748yo.pdf.

———. 2013a. 'Bhutan Poverty Analysis 2012.' Thimphu: National Statistics Bureau, Royal Government of Bhutan. http://www.nsb.gov.bt/publication/files/pub10a-t10635il.pdf.

———. 2013b. '"Key Indicators."'. http://www.nsb.gov.bt/main/indicator.php.

———. 2013c. 'National Statistics Bureau Website.' http://www.nsb.gov.bt

National Traditional Medicine Hospital. 2007. 'National Traditional Medicine Professional Service Standard.' Internal document. Thimphu: National Traditional Medicine Hospital, Royal Government of Bhutan.

———. 2011. *Traditional Medicine Disease Classification*. 2nd ed. Thimphu: National Traditional Medicine Hospital, Royal Government of Bhutan.

Nebesky-Wojkowitz, René de. 1956. *Oracles and Demons of Tibet: The Cult and Iconography of the Tibetan Protective Deities*. The Hague: Mouton.

Nichter, Mark, and Mimi Nichter. 1996. *Anthropology and International Health*. London: Routledge.

Nidup, Dorji. 2009. 'Les Nga: Traditional Therapy Procedures.' *Menjong Sorig Journal* (2): 11–16.

———. 2010. 'The Concepts of gSo.Ba-Rig.Pa.' *Menjong Sorig Journal* (3): 1–11.

Office of the Census Commissioner. 2005. 'Results of the Population and Housing Census of Bhutan.' Thimphu: Office of the Census Commissioner, Royal Government of Bhutan. http://www.bhutancensus.gov.bt.

Ohnuki-Tierney, Emiko. 1984. *Illness and Culture in Contemporary Japan: An Anthropological View*. Cambridge: Cambridge University Press.

Okely, Judith. 1999. 'Love, Care and Diagnosis.' In *Extending the Boundaries of Care: Medical Ethics and Caring Practices*, ed. Tamara Kohn and Rosemary McKechnie, 19–48. Oxford: Berg Publishers.

Ong, Aihwa. 2005. 'Ecologies of Expertise: Assembling Flows, Managing Citizenship.' In *Global Assemblages: Technology, Politics, and Ethics as Anthropological Problems*, ed. Stephen J. Collier and Aihwa Ong. Oxford: Wiley-Blackwell.

Ong, Aihwa, and Stephen J. Collier. 2004a. 'Global Assemblages, Anthropological Problems.' In *Global Assemblages: Technology, Politics, and Ethics as Anthropological Problems*, ed. Aihwa Ong and Stephen J. Collier. Oxford: Wiley-Blackwell.

———. (ed.). 2004b. *Global Assemblages: Technology, Politics, and Ethics as Anthropological Problems*. Oxford: Wiley-Blackwell.

Pain, Adam. 2004. 'State, Economy and Space in Bhutan in the Early Part of 19th Century.' In *The Spider and the Piglet: Proceedings of the First International Seminar on Bhutan Studies*, ed. Karma Ura and Sonam Kinga, 160–93. Thimphu: Centre for Bhutan Studies.

Pedey, Karma. 2005. *Ta She Gha Chha: The Broken Saddle and Other Popular Bhutanese Beliefs*. Thimphu: DSB Publication.

Pelden, Sonam. 2012a. 'Understanding Drug Shortage.' *Kuensel* Online, 12 January. http://www.kuenselonline.com/2011/?p=24957.

Pelden, Sonam. 2012b. 'Traditional Healers Soar at 1,683.' *Kuensel* Online, 13 February. http://www.kuenselonline.com/2011/?p=26984.

Pelgen, Ugyen. 2000. 'Karamshing: An Antidote against Evil.' In *New Horizons in Bon Studies*, ed. S. Karmay and Y. Nagano, 671–83. Bon Studies 2, Senri Ethnological Reports. Osaka: National Museum of Ethnology.

Pem, Tandin. 2011. 'Monk Gets Three Years for Smuggling Tobacco.' *Bhutan Observer*, 3 April, online edition. http://bhutanobserver.bt/3744-bo-news-about-monk_gets_three_years_for_smuggling_tobacco_.aspx.

Petryna, Adriana. 2002. *Life Exposed: Biological Citizens after Chernobyl*. Princeton, NJ: Princeton University Press.

Petryna, Adriana, and Arthur Kleinman. 2006. 'The Pharmaceutical Nexus.' In *Global Pharmaceuticals: Ethics, Markets, Practices*, ed. Adriana Petryna, Andrew Lakoff, and Arthur Kleinman, 1–32. Durham, NC: Duke University Press.

Petryna, Adriana, Andrew Lakoff, and Arthur Kleinman (ed.). 2006. *Global Pharmaceuticals: Ethics, Markets, Practices*. Durham, NC: Duke University Press.

Phuntsho, Karma. 2004. 'Echoes of Ancient Ethos: Reflections on Some Popular Bhutanese Social Themes.' In *The Spider and the Piglet: Proceedings of the First International Seminar on Bhutan Studies*, ed. Karma Ura and Sonam Kinga, 564–80. Thimphu: Centre for Bhutan Studies.

———. 2013. *The History of Bhutan*. New Delhi: Random House, India.

Pommaret, Françoise. 2004. 'Yul and Yul Lha: The Territory and Its Deity in Bhutan.' Bulletin of Tibetology, Gangtok: Namgyal Institute of Tibetology 40 (1) (May): 39–67.

———. 2009. '"Local Community Rituals" in Bhutan: Documentation and Tentative Reading.' In *Buddhism Beyond the Monastery: Tantric Practices and Their Performers in Tibet and the Himalayas*, ed. Sarah Jacoby and Antonio Terrone. Leiden: Brill.

Pordié, Laurent (ed.). 2012. *Tibetan Medicine in the Contemporary World: Global Politics of Medical Knowledge and Practice*. London: Routledge.

Post, Stephen G. 2000. *The Moral Challenge of Alzheimer Disease: Ethical Issues from Diagnosis to Dying*. Baltimore: JHU Press.

Prost, Audrey. 2008. *Precious Pills: Medicine and Social Change among Tibetan Refugees in India*. Epistemologies of Healing. New York: Berghahn Books.

Rabinow, Paul, and Nikolas Rose. 2006. 'Biopower Today.' *BioSocieties* 1(2) (June): 195–217. doi:10.1017/S1745855206040014.

Ramphel, Norbu. 1999. *Bhutan through the Ages*. 3 vols. New Delhi: Anmol Publications Pvt. Ltd.

Reig, José Luis Peset, and Diego Gracia. 1992. *The Ethics of Diagnosis*. New York: Springer.

Ren, Yegang. 2007. 'Is TV Changing Bhutan?' *China's Ethnic Groups* 5(3): 46–49.

Rennie, D. F. 1866. *Bhotan and the Story of the Dooar War*. London: J. Murray.

Rennie, Frank, and Robin Mason (eds.). 2008. *Bhutan: Ways of Knowing*. Charlotte, NC: Information Age Publishing.

Rinpoche Rechung. 1973. *Tibetan Medicine: Illustrated in Original Texts*. Berkeley: University of California Press.

Rose, Nikolas, and Peter Miller. 1992. 'Political Power beyond the State: Problematics of Government.' *British Journal of Sociology* 43(2) (1 June): 173–205. doi:10.2307/591464.

Rose, Nikolas, and Carlos Novas. 2008. 'Biological Citizenship.' In *Global Assemblages*, ed. Aihwa Ong and Stephen J. Collier, 439–463. Oxford: Blackwell Publishing Ltd. http://onlinelibrary.wiley.com/doi/10.1002/9780470696569.ch23/summary.

Royal Government of Bhutan. 1995. 'Forest and Nature Conservation Act of Bhutan.'
———. 2004. 'Penal Code of Bhutan.' https://www.unodc.org/tldb/pdf/Bhutan_Penal_ Code_2004_Eng.pdf.
———. 2008. 'Constitution of the Kingdom of Bhutan.'
Saillant, Francine, and Serge Genest. 2006. *Medical Anthropology: Regional Perspectives and Shared Concerns*. Malden: Wiley.
Samuel, Geoffrey. 1993. *Civilized Shamans: Buddhism in Tibetan Societies*. Washington, DC: Smithsonian Institution Press.
———. 2001. 'Tibetan Medicine in Contemporary India: Theory and Practice.' In *Healing Powers and Modernity: Traditional Medicine, Shamanism, and Science in Asian Societies*, ed. Linda Connor and Geoffrey Samuel, 247–68. Westport, CT: Bergin & Garvey.
Samuel, Geoffrey, and Cathy Cantwell. Forthcoming. *The Seed of Immortal Life: Contexts and Meanings of a Tibetan Longevity Practice*. Kathmandu: Vajra Books.
Saxer, Martin. 2010. 'Manufacturing Tibetan Medicine: The Creation of an Industry and Moral Economy of Tibetanness.' PhD thesis. Oxford: University of Oxford.
Scheper-Hughes, Nancy, and Margaret M. Lock. 1987. 'The Mindful Body: A Prolegomenon to Future Work in Medical Anthropology.' *Medical Anthropology Quarterly* 1(1) (1 March): 6–41. doi:10.2307/648769.
Schrempf, Mona. 2007. 'Bon Lineage Doctors and the Local Transmission of Knowing Medical Practice in Nagchu.' In *Soundings in Tibetan Medicine: Anthropological and Historical Perspectives: PIATS 2003: Tibetan Studies: Proceedings of the Tenth Seminar of the International Association for Tibetan Studies, Oxford, 2003*, ed. Mona Schrempf, 91–126. Brill.
———. 2015a. 'Spider, Soul, and Healing in Eastern Bhutan'. In *Festschrift for Per Kvaerne*, ed. Hanna Havnevik and Charles Ramble, 481–97. Oslo: The Institute for Comparative Research in Human Culture.
———. 2015b. 'Fighting Illness with Gesar: A Healing Ritual from Eastern Bhutan.' In *Tibetan and Himalayan Healing: An Anthology for Anthony Aris*, ed. Charles Ramble and Ulrike Rösler, 621–30. Oxford: Oxford University Press.
———. 2015c. 'Becoming a Female Ritual Healer in East Bhutan.' In *Women as Visionaries, Healers and Agents of Social Transformation – Female Religious Specialists between Autonomy and Ambivalence in Tibet, the Himalayas and Inner Asia, Revue d'Etudes Tibétaines*, (special issue), ed. M. Schrempf and N. Schneider. 34 (Décembre 2015), 189–213.
Selin, Helaine (ed.). 2003. *Medicine across Cultures: History and Practice of Medicine in Non-Western Cultures*. Dordrecht: Kluwer Academic Publishers.
Sharma, Ursula. 1992. *Complementary Medicine Today: Practitioners and Patients*. London: Routledge.
Shim, Janet, Sharon Kaufman, and Ann Russ. 2007. 'Clinical Life: Expectation and the Double Edge of Medical Promise.' *Health* 11(2) (1 April): 245–64. doi:10.1177/1363459307074696.
———. 2009. 'Aged Bodies and Kinship Matters: The Ethical Field of Kidney Transplant.' In *Social Bodies*, ed. Helen Lambert and Maryon McDonald, 17–46. New York: Berghahn Books.
Sidhu, Pushpinder, and Hugh O. O'Kane. 2001. 'Self-Managed Anticoagulation: Results from a Two-Year Prospective Randomized Trial with Heart Valve Patients.' *Annals of Thoracic Surgery* 72(5) (November): 1523–27. doi:10.1016/S0003-4975(01)03049-1.
Siebert, S. F., and J. M. Belsky. 2007. 'Reflections on Conservation Education and Practice in Bhutan.' *Journal of Bhutan Studies*, 16:83–111.

Siena, Kevin Patrick. 2005. *Sins of the Flesh: Responding to Sexual Disease in Early Modern Europe.* Toronto: Centre for Reformation and Renaissance Studies.

Singer, Merrill, and Hans Baer. 2011. *Introducing Medical Anthropology: A Discipline in Action.* Lanham, MD: Rowman Altamira.

Singer, Merrill, and Pamela I. Erickson. 2011. *A Companion to Medical Anthropology.* Chichester: John Wiley & Sons.

Singh, Nagendra. 1978. *Bhutan: A Kingdom in the Himalayas; A Study of the Land, Its People, and Their Government.* New Delhi: Thomson Press Publication Division.

Singha, Komol. 2013. 'Tourism, Environment and Economic Growth in Himalayan Kingdom of Bhutan.' In *Knowledge Systems of Societies for Adaptation and Mitigation of Impacts of Climate Change,* ed. Sunil Nautiyal, K. S. Rao, Harald Kaechele, K. V. Raju, and Ruediger Schaldach, 651–67. Berlin: Environmental Science and Engineering. Springer Berlin Heidelberg.

Singye, Jigme. 2012. 'Study of the Efficacy of Hot Compression.' *Menjong Sorig Journal* (5): 116–28.

Stafford, Lindsay. 2011. 'WHO Developing New Traditional Medicine Classification.' *Herbal E Gram,* 8(1). Austin: American Botanical Council

Stokowski, Laura A. 2006. 'Fundamentals of Phototherapy for Neonatal Jaundice.' *Advances in Neonatal Care: Official Journal of the National Association of Neonatal Nurses* 6 (6) (December): 303–12. doi:10.1016/j.adnc.2006.08.004.

Stoner, Bradley P. 1986. 'Understanding Medical Systems: Traditional, Modern, and Syncretic Health Care Alternatives in Medically Pluralistic Societies.' *Medical Anthropology Quarterly* 17 (2) (February): 44–48.

Strathern, Andrew, and Pamela J. Stewart. 2010. *Curing and Healing: Medical Anthropology in Global Perspective.* Durham, NC: Carolina Academic Press.

Strathern, Marilyn. 1990. *The Gender of the Gift.* Berkeley: University of California Press.

———. 1992. 'Parts and Wholes: Refiguring Relationships in a Postplural World.' In *Conceptualizing Society,* ed. Adam Kuper. London: Routledge.

Tashi, Khenpo Phuntsho. 2005. 'The Positive Impact on Gomchen Tradition on Achieving and Maintaining Gross National Happiness.' In *Rethinking Development: Local Pathways to Global Wellbeing.* Antigonish: St. Francis Xavier University.

Tashi, Tshering. 2009. 'From Byways to a Highway.' In *From Jesuits to Jetsetters Bold Bhutan Beckons: Inhaling Gross National Happiness,* 184–222. Brisbane: Copyright Pub. Co.

Tenzin, Sherab. 2008. 'Collection of Medicinal Plants and the Production of Traditional Medicines in Bhutan.' *Menjong Sorig Journal* (1): 63–69.

The Bhutanese. 2012. 'Three Crises That Created the Rupee Crisis.' *The Bhutanese,* 18 April. http://www.thebhutanese.bt/three-crises-that-created-the-rupee-crisis/.

Tidy, Colin. 2010. 'Neonatal Jaundice.' Patient.co.uk. http://www.patient.co.uk/doctor/neonatal-jaundice.

Trashi, Tshering. 2010a. 'The Chagpori Healers: Part 1.' *Kuensel.* http://www.kuenselonline.com/modules.php?name=News&file=article&sid=16190.

———. 2010b. 'The Chagpori Healers: Part 2.' *Kuensel.* http://www.kuenselonline.com/modules.php?name=News&file=article&sid=16271.

Tsarong, T. J. 1981. *Fundementals of Tibetan Medicine according to the Rgyud-Bzhi.* Ed. J. G. Drakton and L. Chomphei. Trans. J. G. Drakton. Dharamsala: Tibetan Medical Center.

Tshering, Dechen, Tempa Wangdi, and Thinley Zangmo. 2013. 'Traditional Healers: Quacks or Miracle Curers?' *Kuensel* Online, 28 August. http://www.kuenselonline.com/ktwosection/traditional-healers-quacks-or-miracle-curers/#.UjIsVry8pQW.

Tshering, K. 2009. 'Agriculture and Usage of Natural Resources in Bhutan.' *Journal of the Faculty of Agriculture, Shinshu University* 45(1–2): 33–42. CABDirect2.

Turner, Edith. 2011. *Experiencing Ritual: A New Interpretation of African Healing.* Philadelphia: University of Pennsylvania Press.

Turner, Victor. 1957. *Schism and Continuity in an African Society: A Study of Ndembu Village Life.* Manchester: Manchester University Press for the Rhodes-Livingstone Institute, Northern Rhodesia.

———. 1962. *Chihamba, the White Spirit: A Ritual Drama of the Ndembu.* Vol. 33. The Rhodes-Livingstone Papers. Manchester and New York: Published on behalf of the Rhodes-Livingstone Institute by the Manchester University Press; Humanities Press.

———. 1967. *The Forest of Symbols: Aspects of Ndembu Ritual.* Ithaca, NY: Cornell University Press.

Ulmasova, Sabrina. 2013. 'The Hydro-Electrical Power Sector in Bhutan: An Economic Assessment.' MA thesis. Kingston: University of Rhode Island. http://www.edc.uri.edu/mesm/Docs/MajorPapers/Ulmasova_2013.pdf.

United Nations. 2013. 'Solution Exchange Bhutan.' http://www.solutionexchange-un.net.bt/bhutan/.

United States Pharmacopeia Convention. 2013. *The United States Pharmacopeia: The National Formulary.* United States Pharmacopeial Convention, Incorporated.

Upadhyay, B. N. 2000. *From Mountain Kingdom to Public Sector.* Delhi: Devika Publications.

Ura, Karma. 1994. 'Development and Decentralisation in Medieval and Modern Bhutan.' In *Bhutan: Aspects of Culture and Development,* ed. Michael Aris and Michael Hutt, 25–49. Kiscadale Asia Research Series no. 5. Gartmore: Kiscadale.

———. 2002. 'Perceptions of Security.' *South Asian Security: Futures.* Colombo: Regional Centre for Strategic Studies, Sri Lanka: 59–79.

———. 2009a. 'A Proposal for GNH Value Education in Schools.' Thimphu: Gross National Happiness Commission

———. 2009b. 'Gross National Happiness as a Larger Context for Healing and Global Change.' Paper presented at the ICTAM VII Seventh International Congress Traditional Asian Medicine, Thimphu, Bhutan.

———. 2009c. 'The Bhutanese Development Story.' *Monograph Series* 15. Thimphu: Centre for Bhutan Studies.

Ura, Karma, and Sonam Kinga (eds.). 2004. *The Spider and the Piglet: Proceedings of the First International Seminar on Bhutan Studies.* Thimphu: Centre for Bhutan Studies.

Ura, Karma, and Dorji Penjore (eds.). 2009. *Gross National Happiness: Practice and Measurement.* Thimphu: Centre for Bhutan Studies.

Walcott, Susan M. 2011. 'One of a Kind: Bhutan and the Modernity Challenge.' *National Identities* 13(3): 253–65. doi:10.1080/14608944.2011.585633.

Wangchuk, Dasho Sangay. 2008. 'Culture and Bhutan.' In *Bhutan: Ways of Knowing,* ed. Frank Rennie and Robin Mason, 61–64. Charlotte, NC: Information Age Publishing.

Wangchuk, Dorji. 2008. 'Traditional Medicine in Bhutan.' *Menjong Sorig Journal* (1): 75–93.

———. 2010. 'Prevention of Age Related Diseases through the Application of gSo-Ba Rig-Pa Wisdom and Products.' *Menjong Sorig Journal* (3): 12–25.

Wangchuk, Kinga. 2008. 'Search for Insect Fungi Leads to the Discovery of New Species of Cordyceps from Gedu Forest.' *Menjong Sorig Journal* (1): 99–102.

Wangchuk, Phurpa. 2008. 'Health Impacts of Traditional Medicines and Bio-prospecting: A World Scenario Accentuating Bhutan's Perspective.' *Journal of Bhutan Studies* 18, 116–134 .

Wangchuk, Phurpa. 2009. 'Bio-prospecting in Bhutan: Its Scope and Challenges.' *Menjong Sorig Journal* (2): 39–45.

———. 2010. 'A Search for Goji Berry-Lycium Barbarum in Bhutan and Its Relative.' *Menjong Sorig Journal* (3): 50–57.

Wangchuk, Phurpa, Paul A. Keller, Stephen G. Pyne, Thanapat Sastraruji, Malai Taweechotipatr, Roonglawan Rattanajak, Aunchalee Tonsomboon, and Sumalee Kamchonwongpaisan. 2012. 'Phytochemical and Biological Activity Studies of the Bhutanese Medicinal Plant Corydalis Crispa.' *Natural Product Communications* 7(5) (May): 575–80.

Wangchuk, Phurpa, Dorji Wangchuk, and Jens Aagaard-Hansen. 2007. 'Traditional Bhutanese Medicine (gSo-BA Rig-PA): An Integrated Part of the Formal Health Care Services.' *Southeast Asian Journal of Tropical Medicine and Public Health* 38(1) (January): 161–67.

Wangchuk, Tshering. 2009. 'Golden Needle Therapy (Serkhap).' *Menjong Sorig Journal* (2): 56–59.

Wangdi, Tempa. 2011. '"Dangerous" Indigenous Healers Thrive Despite Modern Hospitals.' *Bhutan Observer*, 26 March, online edition. http://bhutanobserver.bt/3916-bo-news-about-dangerous_indigenous_healers_thrive_despite_modern_hospitals_.aspx.

Wangdi, Tendril. 2008. 'Blood Letting and the Cauterization in Bhutanese Traditional Medicine.' *Menjong Sorig Journal* (1): 133–46.

Wangmo, Chime. 1985. 'Rituals of Bhutanese House Construction in Bhutan.' In *Soundings in Tibetan Civilization*, ed. B. Aziz and M. Kapstein, 107–14. New Delhi: Manohar.

Wangmo, Neyzang, Simon David Barraclough, and Beverley Wood. 2007. 'Development of Nursing in Bhutan: An Overview.' *Asian Journal of Nursing* 10(3): 148–55.

Wangmo, Tashi. 2012. 'Rupee Crunch Exacerbates Drug Shortage.' *The Bhutanese*, 18 April. http://www.thebhutanese.bt/rupee-crunch-exacerbates-drug-shortage/.

Wangyal, Tashi. 2001. 'Ensuring Social Sustainability: Can Bhutan's Education System Ensure Intergenerational Transmission of Values?' *Journal of Bhutan Studies* 3(1): 106–31.

Ward, Michael, and Frederic Jackson. 1965. 'Medicine in Bhutan.' *Lancet* 285 (7389) (10 April): 811–13. doi:10.1016/S0140-6736(65)92976-4.

Weber, Max. 1997. *The Theory of Social and Economic Organization*. New York: Simon and Schuster.

White, J. C. 1984. *Sikkim and Bhutan*. Leiden: Brill.

Whitecross, Richard. 2004. 'The Thrimzhung Chenmo and the Emergence of Contemporary Bhutanese Legal System.' In *The Spider and the Piglet: Proceedings of the First International Seminar on Bhutan Studies*, ed. Karma Ura and Sonam Kinga, 355–78. Thimphu: Centre for Bhutan Studies.

World Health Organization. 2008. 'WHO: Traditional Medicine.' Website December. http://www.who.int/medicines/areas/traditional/en/

———. 2010. 'WHO to Define Information Standards for Traditional Medicine.' 7 December 2010. http://www.who.int/mediacentre/news/notes/2010/trad_medicine_20101207/en/index.html.

Wikan, Unni, and Fredrik Barth. 2011. *Situation of Children in Bhutan: An Anthropological Perspective*. Thimphu: Centre for Bhutan Studies.

Wilson, Thomas M., and Hastings Donnan. 1998. *Border Identities: Nation and State at International Frontiers*. Cambridge: Cambridge University Press.

Winkler, Daniel. 2008. 'Yartsa Gunbu (Cordyceps Sinensis) and the Fungal Commodification of Tibet's Rural Economy.' *Economic Botany* 62(3) (1 November): 291–305. doi:10.1007/s12231-008-9038-3.

Witt, Claudia M., Nadine E. J. Berling, Ngari Thingo Rinpoche, Mingji Cuomo, and Stefan N. Willich. 2009. 'Evaluation of Medicinal Plants as Part of Tibetan Medicine Prospective Observational Study in Sikkim and Nepal.' *Journal of Alternative and Complementary Medicine* 15(1) (January): 59–65. doi:10.1089/acm.2008.0176.

World Bank. 2015. 'Data: Bhutan.' http://data.worldbank.org/country/bhutan.

Xu, Jianchu, R. Edward Grumbine, Arun Shrestha, Mats Eriksson, Xuefei Yang, Yun Wang, and Andreas Wilkes. 2009. 'Las Himalaya Se Derriten: Efectos En Cascada Del Cambio Climático Sobre El Agua, La Biodiversidad y Los Medios de Vida.' *Conservation Biology* 23(3): 520–30. doi:10.1111/j.1523-1739.2009.01237.x.

Yangka. 2008. 'A Bhutanese Learning Abroad.' In *Bhutan: Ways of Knowing*, ed. Frank Rennie and Robin Mason, 7–12. Charlotte, NC: Information Age Publishing.

Index